THE
COMPLEAT
PHYSICIAN

REFLECTIONS FROM A GOLDEN AGE OF CLINICAL MEDICINE

DENIS R BENJAMIN
B.SC., M.B.,B.CH.

Library-of-Congress Cataloguing-in-Publication Data

ISBN 978-0-9829359-2-7 (Paperback)

Benjamin, Denis R.

1.Medical School - Education - Pathologist - South Africa- Johannesburg - Seattle

First edition 2019
Published by Tembe Publishing, Fort Worth, TX, USA. Printed in the United States of America.

Dedicated to teachers
of clinical medicine

"We are told that stories are living beings,
they grow, they develop, they remember,
they change not in their essence, but
sometimes in their dress."
(*Braiding Sweetgrass: Indigenous Wisdom,
Scientific Knowledge and the Teachings of
Plants* -Robin Wall Kimmerer)

CONTENTS

Prologue

All these chronicles are true, at least in essence. Some of the events occurred over fifty years ago. The stories have been recounted so often that some details may have become embellished, polished or perhaps distorted. But they are as vivid as when they occurred.

They begin at the University of Witwatersrand in Johannesburg, South Africa in the 1960s, and then move to the University of Washington in Seattle, USA, a decade later. Two time periods and two worlds apart. Seattle was about as far away from my home as one could travel for additional medical training. I might have considered Alaska, but it still does not have a medical school. The stories cover life at medical school, the travails of internships and residency and the early days of medical practice. It is also the saga of immigration and the adoption of a new country. It follows the Darwinian principle for survival - move, adapt or perish.

To appreciate the context, recall the state of the world at the time, especially South Africa. The

Republic of South Africa 1960s — world pariah. International economic sanctions. Banned from participation in the Olympic games. The apartheid system is in full force, but small cracks are appearing. The Black Sash movement, spearheaded by a group of courageous women, led to frequent street protests. The Sharpeville massacre, during which 69 black protesters were killed and hundreds wounded, greeted the decade, and was still a fresh memory for all of us, as well as a permanent scar on our psyches. One doesn't easily forget photographs of dozens of innocent people shot in the back. Nelson Mandela was imprisoned in 1962. No one thought he would ever step off Robben Island. The national universities were still accepting a few non-white students, although this soon ceased, forcing those who wished to become physicians into the segregated university in Durban. The apartheid system seemed entrenched. Immutable.

It was in this milieu that we rushed to the offices of the morning newspaper, the Rand Daily Mail, located in the center of Johannesburg. It published the results of our high school matriculation examinations. Our entire fate was in the balance. Futures depended on a few words — pass, fail, and the number of "distinctions" — those subjects in which one might have excelled, but which the examiners were very stingy in awarding. The matriculation results were posted on boards pasted on the outside wall of the building. They were printed alphabetically in small font. One had to get very close to read them. We swarmed into the street, pushing and shoving to the front. This culminated with screams of delight or cries of anguish.

Unlike in many other countries or later times, acceptance into medical school was entirely dependent on this one examination. No essays, no donations to the alumni association or the football program, no nepotism, no bribery, no long list of nonprofit organizations for which one had volunteered. The rule was simple and brutal. The higher one's result in this single final matriculation examination — plus any distinctions, especially mathematics, science or Latin — the better. Nothing else mattered. No negotiation. No claiming any special privilege. No filing a court case suggesting some form of discrimination. Unfortunately, the less privileged in the society, comprising over eighty percent of the general population, were largely excluded from this system. Most never even had the opportunity to compete, and for those that did, the number of available positions was very limited.

The discrimination for acceptance into medical school was not limited to race alone. Women, too, faced significant challenges. In part this was a reflection of the time and the expectations. There were few female-physician role models. Many of the all-girl schools did not even offer Latin or some of the sciences as part of their curriculum. They offered biology, at that time a "soft" science, but not physics or chemistry. There was still the widespread societal stereotype of male doctors and female nurses. So it is not surprising that the women who broke through this barrier became overachievers, many eclipsing their male colleagues.

I was one of the fortunate, having the right skin color, gender, supportive parents and some brilliant teachers at King Edward VII High School — a public, boys only, white only, English-speaking school. It was typical at the time to be segregated into small discrete groups — your clan. Perhaps the word "egalitarian" was not in the Afrikaans dictionary. Even though my family was firmly entrenched in the middle class — I can only recall a couple of family vacations while growing up — the cost of medical school was not an issue. For all intents and purposes it was free, although the small grant I received from my father's Masonic lodge allowed me to purchase some text books.

Finally, I wriggled my way to the front of the crowd and scanned the B's. I stood there with a sense of relief, about to turn seventeen, knowing I was headed to medical school, and would perhaps one day become a physician.

Chapter 1. Contrasts

Some of the following narratives may not resonate with readers in the United States of America. Starting medical school at seventeen years of age? No electives? No undergraduate degree? Those who grew up in the remnants of the British Empire will find them more familiar, as the colonial British established standard educational, judicial, transportation and political systems in every country they occupied. They even taught everyone cricket, rugby, croquet, lawn bowls and field hockey. Americans rebelled early, creating their own systems. For medical training, following the critical Flexner report in 1910, this involved first getting an undergraduate degree in whatever subjects — although most choose pre-med courses— followed by four years of medical school as graduate students. After this most continue on with residencies in their specialties.

In contrast, training to be a doctor in the British inspired systems begins right out of high school. Being undergraduates we behaved like undergraduates, despite the seriousness of the profession. We were young, debt free, usually still single, and many of us still lived at home. This created a different dynamic and environment compared to the more mature American medical student, who had already completed four years of college, was probably married, already in significant debt, living far from family and friends. Some of the playfulness in our training would be unthinkable within the US system.

The South African/British medical school curriculum had been carefully honed over the centuries. Students did not ask questions about relevance. We expected that what we were learning had some value, even if we could not discern it at the time. The philosophy was to build a firm and broad foundation of essential biological knowledge, constructing the edifice of clinical medicine on top of this base. We knew that we would not see a living patient in the first three years of medical school. New knowledge was incorporated into the curriculum, but wholesale changes were avoided. There were no standing curriculum committees frequently changing the system. The curriculum was designed to produce the best possible doctors to meet societies' and patients' needs. It was not intended to satisfy the

7

whims of a student. Students were there to be moulded, like lumps of clay.

The USA could not have been more different. While there was certainly the intention to produce excellent physicians, much of the curriculum catered to the student's needs and aspirations. This fundamental philosophical difference can't be overstated. These approaches address two different questions — do you want satisfied patients or satisfied students? Most agree that both is the optimal goal, but the two systems tilt in different directions.

Another striking contrast was the expectation for the medical school faculty. In South Africa the faculty were first and foremost physicians, responsible for the care of their patients. Teaching aspiring students was their next priority, which they took very seriously; research and publications, while valued, was at the bottom of the list. In the USA, these priorities are reversed. Many faculty only have clinical responsibilities for a couple of months a year. Research, publications and grant funding dominate their lives. Teaching is often regarded as a necessary evil. It is cruel, albeit well known, that the individual who is voted "teacher of the year" by the students, is very likely to lose their job, implying that they are not spending enough time in the laboratory or writing grant proposals.

For a variety of social and cultural reasons, the general public accepted medical students as an integral component of care in a teaching hospital. Rarely did a patient object. Many procedures were performed by medical students, under the watchful eye of a more senior physician. While this does occur in the USA, especially in the surgical disciplines, under the rubric of "see one—do one—teach one", most of the time medical students are mere observers.

In addition to passing all the examinations, certification and licensing as a doctor required a number of additional requirements, including a minimum number of normal deliveries. We had to administer fifty anesthetics during our internship year, putting the patient to sleep, and more importantly ensuring that they woke up. However the most crucial requirement was the completion of an additional year as a house officer (aka intern), spending six months in general surgery and six months in general medicine in a provincial teaching hospital. This was the time that the newly minted graduates took almost complete responsibility for the care of their patients.

When I began pathology training in the USA, none of my colleagues had this background. They had not developed the skills of communicating with either their medical colleagues or patients. When I joined ward-rounds at the children's hospital to assist my colleagues in selecting the most appropriate laboratory tests or to discuss the results of a biopsy, the general consensus was that Benjamin was crazy. Pathologists had not been seen on the patient floors. Even the university department changed its name from Clinical Pathology to Laboratory Medicine, underscoring that we were not welcome in the clinic.

At the end of six years at medical school, a year of internship, and having all the requirements signed off by the necessary authorities, we received a letter from the South African Medical and Dental Council, certifying that we were now ready to be unleashed on the general public without further supervision. We also received an application for malpractice insurance if wanted, for the princely sum of about $50 a year. At that time it was unnecessary.

Chapter 2. Anatomizing

It was a year before we moved from the main campus of the University of Witwatersrand up to the medical school in Hillbrow. During that time we learned the basic sciences — chemistry, physics, zoology and botany — foundations for the future. Only then were we deemed to be acceptable student material. It was also known that a many as 10% of first year students would be washed out by the rigors of that year, requiring them to pursue other occupations. This pyramid system was based on the idea — "we give you one chance; you prove that you are worthy."

Wearing pristine, white, laboratory coats we were ushered into the anatomy department and the Vesalian dissection halls. Each of us had chosen a partner with whom we would spend the entire year disassembling a pickled corpse, learning human anatomy. On the other side of each dissection table was another twosome — selected at random. Our companions were physiotherapy students who underwent the identical anatomy training. I remember the name of one, but not the other, primarily because of the legacy of her parents. The family name was Healing and her parents, in all their wisdom, named her Faith.

We stood at attention at our assigned table. A member of the clergy whose denomination was a mystery conducted a service of sorts, commemorating the collective lives and deaths of the departed. We began adapting to the reek of formalin, an odor that would infiltrate our clothes and skin for the coming year. The service was somber and moving. Professor Philip Tobias, the chairman of the Anatomy Department then recounted the history of human anatomizing, the privilege that was being bestowed on us, and the sacredness of the moment.

At the end of the ceremony we unwrapped our cadaver for the first time. For most, this was our initial introduction to death. The naked porcelain on the dissection table was surreal. The body was accompanied by a brief description, such as age, weight, cause of death, other diseases etc, but no mention of a family, a job, or any fragment of his or her life. At the same time, this helped to separate us from the fact that this once was a living person.

During the first few weeks we got to know our cadaver with some intimacy. But we were still children, and kids will be kids. It did not take long before the intense seriousness departed. Casualness replaced the sense of awe. It began one evening. We all worked at different paces, so the dissection halls were kept open one evening a week — a chance to catch up if one had fallen behind. A group of us used this opportunity to have dinner together, and then spend the night exposing the next layer of muscle. The problem occurred when our entire dinner was consumed in a nearby pub and was mainly liquid, consisting of two carbon fragments. The combination of alcohol and testosterone sometimes leads to mean-spirited adventures.

One of our colleagues lacked any sense of humor. We decided that it might be amusing to watch her reaction the next day when unwrapping her cadaver she discovered that its was not her cadaver. So we moved some bodies — after all, that is what friends are for. The event was whispered around the dissection hall the next morning, knowing that she always arrived late with daunting passion and intensity. She rushed in, late as usual, and took the covers and cloth off her corpse. The scream when she

13

saw the face was ear shattering. While she was in the throws of a conniption some-one noted that Professor Tobias, the department chairman, was coming down the hallway and about the enter the dissection hall. Had this prank been discovered it would have meant the premature death of my medical career. Such behavior was a cardinal and unforgivable sin. Realizing the potential explosiveness of the situation, a classmate immediately went into the hallway, distracting the professor by asking some arcane question about the anatomy of a wrist bone. This was enough time to delay his entry. We switched the bodies back, calmed the student down, apologized profusely and led her through a back door into an adjacent room to recover from both the shock and the humiliation. None of us were proud of this escapade, and we never tried anything similar again. However, with the passing of time and the familiarity with death, a definite casualness crept into the dissection halls.

There was a long-held tradition that we refused to forgo. When the time came for a close examination of the genitalia, it was accepted practice that the few females in the class would be given the privilege/task/pleasure of skinning the male organ, exposing the underlying tissues. This was accompanied by chants, moans and various expressions of pain from the watching males. In today's society, such behavior would be grounds for harassment and intimidation. It would not just be frowned upon — it would be expressly prohibited. I suspect that even back then it was not acceptable, but a blind eye was turned from centuries of custom.

The value of our high school Latin education came into sharp focus during anatomy. The names of most body parts and locations are derived from Latin roots. One muscle in particular became a favorite to recite. A friend used this to advantage one evening. He was dating a young woman with a strong religious background and was invited to a family dinner. As the family gathered around the table, the father leaned over to his daughter and said, "Perhaps your friend would like to say grace." Without blinking an eye, he intoned, *"levator labii superioris alaeque nasi."* In awe of his erudition, the family responded with a vigorous 'Amen'. The name of this muscle, roughly translated from the Latin, means the "lifter of the upper lip and the wing of the nose." It is very prominent in horses, allowing them to flare their nostrils.

Mnemonics was a venerated technique in learning anatomy. Generations of preceding medical students had developed numerous devices to retain and regurgitate the immense amount of information embedded in *Gray's Human Anatomy*. As it was expected that we would be familiar with every last detail, many of us relied on mnemonics for help. And the more obscene the better. Perhaps the most famous and well known is the mnemonic for the twelve cranial nerves, which began with — *Oh, oh, oh to touch and feel* — and then became particularly raunchy. The alternative mnemonic was much less memorable - *On old Olympus' towering top a Finn and German viewed some hops.* (Olfactory nerve, Optic nerve, Oculomotor nerve,Trochlear nerve, Trigeminal nerve, Abducens nerve, Facial nerve, Vestibulocochlear nerve, Glossopharyngeal nerve, Vagus nerve, (Spinal) Accessory nerve, Hypoglossal nerve).

Almost all anatomy learning was hands-on — a tactile, olfactory and visual affair, as we painstakingly peeled away each layer of tissue, like an onion. This was coupled with detailed embryology — the only way to understand the complexities of the gut, or how the testes landed up where they do, or how a simple tube becomes remodeled into a four chambered heart. Instruction was provided by the cadaver, a few classic books such as *Gray's Anatomy*, and a scattering of recently graduated physicians who were pursuing a career in surgery. Known as "table doc's" they supervised medical students in their efforts. It was an opportunity for the budding surgeons to hone their knowledge of human anatomy before being unleashed on living human flesh.

And this is how we all learn. As someone stated in the *Lancet* many years ago. "We learn medicine the same way we learn about sex. Whispered comments from those who are only marginally more experienced than we are."

Chapter 3 - Digging for bones

In 1924 the world of paleoanthropology was overturned when Raymond Dart discovered a small skull near Taung, a tiny and unremarkable place north of Johannesburg. An Australian by birth, Dart was coerced to become the first chairman of anatomy at the University of Witwatersrand. He surmised that this childlike skull might be a possible precursor of hominids, perhaps an early or a distant relative of our family. It validated the old Latin phrase - *ex Africa semper aliquod novi* (out of Africa always something new). This event influenced the Anatomy Department and most of its faculty for the next couple of generations, as it evolved into an epicenter for the study of human evolution.

Students were recruited to provide needed muscle and a little intellect for the excavations at a number of sites scattered across what was then called Transvaal, now known as Gauteng. I spent one of my vacations excavating in the area of Makapansgat in northern Transvaal. It was a memorable month. On my arrival, a pet python was moved from my hut to another abode for safekeeping. One morning, when I climbed to the major cave, a beautiful leopard occupied the entry, calmly surveying the country side for its next dinner. I decided that it was not going to be me, and did a slow, deliberate backwards walk, while never making eye contact with the animal. My heart rate soared into the upper hundreds as I backed down the hill.

One of the full-time paleo-anthropologists who spent his days making assumptions and conclusions on a minimum of evidence — as some anthropologists are wont to do — had a disease known as narcolepsy. This is an unfortunate and miserable condition. The victim suddenly and unexpectedly falls asleep. But more than that, they exhibit catalepsy, during which they are completely atonic. Normally this occurs to all of us during REM sleep. An additional problem was that this particular individual enjoyed smoking a pipe, and we had to be vigilant that he did not catch on fire. Even so, the leather vest he wore was covered in burn holes wherever tobacco embers had landed during one of his atonic spells. He attempted to control his symptoms with heroic quantities of tea, so freshly brewed tea was always available, even in the bush.

The excavations were tedious and painstaking, sifting through mountains of sifted sand, pebbles and rocks for something that looked slightly out of place. I did not have much patience for this sort of work, and I failed to document the location of each find with any precision — a fact that did not go unnoticed when I turned in my report at the end of the month. It earned a stern reprimand from Professor Philip Tobias, though he never gave up on me.

Notwithstanding the tedium of poring through dirt each day, it was an incredible experience. Some of the locals had a sixth sense about where to dig, based on careful observation of the plants, soils and geology. None of them had any schooling, but their connection with the land and their exquisite powers of observation made them an invaluable resource. It was my introduction to bio-geography and the relationship of plants to the underlying geology, a subject I returned to four decades later.

The University and the Institute for the Study of Man in Africa which sponsored these excavations, relied on the local workforce for the real muscle. In order to avoid offending and alienating the farmers in the area, we complied with their long established traditional rules for farm labor. This included starting work at daybreak, a time at which I was not at my prime. Every morning I struggled to get to the dig in time to greet the staff.

Another of the anthropologists had a little side gig collecting scorpions for a pharmaceutical company. Evidently they were investigating the potential medical value of the venom extracted from the tail. Whenever a worker turned over a rock exposing a scorpion, this anthropologist strolled over, casually shoveling the arachnid onto his hand. Snakes and scorpions are rightfully regarded with great suspicion by the locals. Having someone pick them up, was clearly the work of the devil. They viewed this anthropologist with a mixture of fear and veneration. He clearly had their attention whenever he made any requests.

With the department's interest in anthropology, it had collected numerous masks of faces from tribes/ groups/clans all across Africa. I was never told how living subjects were convinced to lie still with a straw in each nostril, while their faces were covered with Plaster of Paris. When dry, this was peeled off, acting as a mold for the final face mask, that was painted to accurately reflect the skin color. Other masks were made from bodies donated to the department. These death masks were displayed on hooks along the longest corridor in the anatomy building — dozens of vacant eyes starring down on the passing parade of students. It was an unnerving sight, especially at night when the building was quiet, and someone would walk down the corridor touching each face so that it wobbled and vibrated for a few minutes as if alive.

Despite rather generous bets no one was ever willing to complete the walk down the entire length of the corridor in the dark — the only proscription being the absence of alcohol.

Chapter 4. Bongo - Bald-headed Chimpanzee

The telephone rang as I was climbing into bed one evening . "Prof. Tobias wants you to come over to the laboratory immediately. They shot and killed a chimpanzee in the zoo this afternoon, and he wants to have photographs of the chimp's chromosomes in the morning newspaper." "You're kidding, right," I responded. "No, this is serious. It's no joke. He wants everyone in the class there and has called in one of the technicians as well." "Ok," I said, "I'll fall for it." I dressed and drove the twenty minutes to medical school, fully expecting to see a couple of inebriated classmates sitting laughing on the front steps. No one was there, but the lights in our small laboratory on the second floor were on, the only illumination in the building.

Two members of the class were missing. "Oh, they have gone to the zoo to collect Bongo's testes," I was informed. The story, as best as we could gather, was that Bongo, an elderly and much beloved zoo attraction had escaped from his cage during his cage cleaning in the afternoon, jumped the enclosure and attacked a woman. All the zoologists were out in the field with the tranquilizer dart-guns, and the only remaining weapon at the zoo was a rifle. End of Bongo. This was sad for a number of reasons. We had all grown up with Bongo. Watching a chimpanzee smoke a packet of Lucky Strike cigarettes a day was amusing for children. He was a major zoo attraction, throwing various objects and excrement at those who taunted him.

Professor Tobias never missed an opportunity to present science to the general public. He was a one man public relations department for the medical school. Here was the perfect chance. Bongo would not have died in vain. He would contribute to our understanding of primate evolution by donating his testes so we could examine his chromosomes. At that time very few primate chromosomes had been studied. These were the early days of cytogenetics. Cell culture had yet to become a standard everyday technique, and so the best way to examine chromosomes was in rapidly dividing cells. The testis is the perfect organ, as sperm are constantly being produced, and one could examine both the meiotic and mitotic diving cells.

Our colleagues arrived an hour later, carefully clutching petri dishes containing fragments of testes in a dilute vinegar solution. We gently teased apart the tubules, placed them on slides, covered them with a thin glass cover slip and mashed them down. The hope was that the dividing cells would rupture, spilling their chromosomes onto the glass. This was followed by a lengthy staining procedure. At one point the slides had to remain in one of the staining baths for quite some time, so Tobias invited us all over to his flat for a midnight snack, and to listen to his collection of classical music. Nobody declined the offer.

When we got back to the laboratory I collected my slides. Much to my consternation, the chromosomes, instead of being deeply and uniformly stained had numerous bands of lighter stain across them. "This is hopeless," I announced. "We will never be able to measure them properly when they look like this." We placed the slides back in the stain until they were uniformly dark. It was another decade before investigators realized that what I had been looking at were groups and cluster of genes. Chromosome banding, as it was then called, became a critical tool in genetics for a number of years. In those early days of cytogenetics, chromosomes were merely neatly arranged by their total length and the length of each arm. None of us had any inkling that those bands meant anything other than unwanted noise. This was my best chance for a Nobel Prize and I blew it. It was when I learned that "you only find what you look for, you only look for what you know."

Once we had the perfect preparation, the technician spent a couple of hours taking photographs. We repaired once again to Tobias' flat for breakfast and watched as the sun rose over the hazy golden mine-dumps of Johannesburg. A few hours later the morning newspaper appeared on the streets with photographs of Bongo's chromosomes. "Beloved chimpanzee aids science," or some such headline.

For obscure reasons I was designated to complete the studies on the chromosomes. Perhaps I volunteered. I wrote over twenty drafts of the results and conclusions. As I had never learned to type, my mother volunteered to produce the manuscripts. Many months later I thought that I had written the perfect scientific paper. By then Tobias was on a sabbatical leave at Oxford University in the United Kingdom. I proudly packed up the manuscript and mailed it off. Weeks later I received his response.

"Your photographs are very good. Recommend that you enlist my research assistant to write the manuscript." Another dozen drafts later he was convinced that it warranted publication. It was accepted by the *South African Journal of Science* and remains the first publication in my curriculum vitae. I still have a copy, and when I read it today I have no clue as to what it was about.

Later that year I presented the findings at a meeting of the South African Association for the Advancement of Science. Despite feeling terrified walking to the podium, I was so well rehearsed I imagined that I was at an Eisteddfod performance. This is a Welsh word for a music or poetry performance, widely used when we were children. These were public on-stage performances parents inflicted on their offspring, at which the parent could gloat or cringe depending on the performance of the child. It was when we were all introduced to competitive art. But this is a digression, although it did prepare us for public performance. As I left the stage after my ten minute tour-de-force, some-one came up to me and commented, "Well Mr. Benjamin, I don't know who you are, but you are obviously a student of Professor Tobias."

It was as if I had an academic stamp of approval on my forehead.

Chapter 5. Explosion

As I was a little younger than most of my classmates, an opportunity presented itself that I felt obliged to pursue. The university offered an additional year of science, before resuming the traditional medical curriculum. Sort of like a year abroad, except this was at home in the confines of small laboratories. Over a dozen of us selected this option at the end of our second year. The bigger decision was which major subjects to pursue. The two choices were anatomy and physiology, or micro-anatomy and biochemistry. The macro or the micro. I opted for the micro.

A significant requirement for the year was the completion of a major research project. In micro-anatomy I tackled the question asking what makes organs stop growing? This required the sacrifice of any number of rats. I used the thyroid gland as the model organ. In the rat it is not a large organ, but I became quite adept at removing either half or the whole gland and having most animals survive my limited surgical prowess. I vaguely recall that I got some interesting results and was able to show that growth was not dependent on the amount of work an organ had to perform. Despite filling in many of the details over subsequent decades, this very fundamental question is still not fully understood.

My biochemistry project involved isolating mitochondria, the energy factories of cells, and determining how they reacted to various hormones. It was tedious, painstaking and frustrating work. Towards the end of the year most of us stayed late in the laboratory every evening in an effort to complete our projects. On one particular night my experiment had totally failed, a regular event to which I had become inured. This was science after all, and it seldom goes according to plan.

As I began again to grind up tissue and fire up the ultracentrifuge in order to separate the minute mitochondria from the rest of the cellular debris, I happened to mention to my laboratory mates about an explosive chemical we made as kids and took to parties as a prank. It was suggested that I show the group how it worked. A simple combination of ammonia and iodine, when mixed in the appropriate amounts, produces ammonium triiodide, a contact explosive when dry. After mixing up the brew I dotted small amounts on pieces of filter paper, placing them in a fume hood to dry. By the end of the evening they had not dried sufficiently to detonate and I was mocked by all in the lab. I poured the remaining sludge into the laboratory sink and slunk home to bed. Not only had I wasted an evening with a failed experiment, but my own friends scoffed at me.

The next morning I arrived in the laboratory and turned the faucet on to rinse a flask. There was a flash, a loud blast and smoke filled the room. The iodine compound had dried overnight in a thin film on the bottom of the large sink and the pressure of the water was enough to cause the explosion. Fragments of the chemical were on the floor, in my hair and on my clothing. The sound of the explosion brought Professor Paul Levy running down the corridor into the lab. He opened the door, and as he stepped in puffs of smoke and crackles emanated from his shoes as he stood on morsels of the compound. Every time I moved small plumes of iodine-scented vapor rose from my clothing.

I had redeemed myself in the eyes of my colleagues, but with the powers that be, not so much.

Chapter 6. Unforgettable characters from the preclinical years

During this golden age of medical education in the 1960s, singling out a few of the most unforgettable characters is not easy. For almost all of them teaching was performance art. The forgettable ones are long forgotten, and there were admittedly a few of them, especially in pathology, which ironically became my chosen specialty.

Human embryology was taught by a remarkable individual, Boris Balinsky. Born in Kiev, Ukraine, he was a full professor by age 28. He emigrated to the United Kingdom for a brief time, and finally South Africa, where he became one of the founders of modern bioscience in the country, including experimental embryology, entomology and electron microscopy.   His book, *An Introduction to Embryology,* remains a classic. His lectures, however, were a challenge. He was not only ambidextrous, but an amazing illustrator. He would face the blackboard with a piece of chalk in each hand and rapidly draw a perfectly symmetrical embryo if needed. Even more disconcerting was when each hand drew a different portion of an embryo. He would also keep talking at the same time, with an accent from the old country. The only way to keep up was to work in pairs, one taking notes, the other trying to reproduce the drawings. After the lecture we would swap our work. These were the days long before copying machines, digital cameras or smartphones.

There was one physiology instructor whose name languishes somewhere in my cortex, but my hippocampus must have failed that day to store it because of informational overload. However what it did store was far more important. It was a lecture that changed my life. It was entitled "How to Make Mistakes." I was already a nascent skeptic, having lived with the lies of government officials and the deceptions of industry. Even so I was not fully prepared for this presentation. He selected a number of research papers from a few of the most prestigious scientific journals and proceeded to demonstrate the mistakes in the research that had been missed by the reviewers and the editors. The errors spanned the spectrum from experimental design, the selection of controls, acquisition bias, statistical analysis, to unfounded assumptions and faulty reasoning. It was a tour-de-force, not just of the fallibility of scientific publication, but a warning to all of us to be vigilant and wary about anything we read. That talk informed my lifelong skepticism, to the point that I refuse to believe anything until I have the opportunity to evaluate and understand the science. Even then it requires that the results are reproducible by others. This has made me quite unpopular with both friends and colleagues, and is one of the reasons I earned my chops as a curmudgeon.

One parasitology lecturer was more legendary than the rest. At the time there was debate about the difference in appearances of various fragments between pork and beef tapeworms. They were easy to identify if one had the worm's head, but patients usually brought in only bits and pieces they discovered wriggling in the toilet bowl, known in scientific jargon as proglottids. He determined to resolve the issue, the old fashioned way. He repaired to the local abattoir, found a nice piece of "measly" pork, ate a few mouthfuls in the form of raw pork tartar, and then began collecting the proglottids, carefully documenting all their features at different stages of development. Once this was done, he got rid of the pork tapeworm and ingested some infected cow. This was very, very basic science.

Paul Levy led the department of physiology of which biochemistry was a major section. His style of teaching bordered on the Socratic. I benefitted from this during the year I spent as a science student between the second and third years of medical school. He was determined that we would not emerge from his tutelage as mere geeks, schooled in how electrons flowed through our body or how we capture and utilize energy. To counter this he established a weekly, two-hour seminar at which one of us had to give an hour long lecture, without notes or slides on any subject other than biochemistry or South Africa. The trick was to find a topic of which he was ignorant. This proved nearly impossible. One of my colleagues gave a brilliant exposition about Beethoven's 5th Symphony. As he concluded with the date of its first performance in Vienna (December 22nd 1808), Levy rocked back on his chair and quietly said, "You are right and it was a cool, cloudy Thursday afternoon."

The choice for my first effort was entitled "The Origin of Life," just the kind of arrogance one expects of a twenty year old. There had been recent experiments demonstrating that electric sparks, simulating lightning, when passed though a mixture of gases postulated to comprise the Earth's atmosphere 400 billion years ago, resulted in the production of organic molecules. What I did not know when I blithely selected this subject was that Professor Levy had recently been elevated to the Department Chair. It was an university tradition that this promotion was always accompanied by a public lecture in the Great Hall of the university. The topic he had chosen was "The Origin of Life." His patience with my presentation was admirable.

My second selection, many months later, was on the creation of obsolescence in the marketplace, based largely on Vance Packard's influential book in the 1960s - *The Waste Makers*. It turned out that Levy was quite aware of this economic perversion dating much earlier to the 1930s, when the auto industry had reached a saturation point and needed new customers.

Lectures in anatomy were sparse, but could be most entertaining, especially those by the head of the department, Phillip Tobias. Few will forget his performance on the difference between human gait and those of the great apes as he leapt onto the lectern to demonstrate. Or the selection of victim classmates to stand in their underwear to illustrate the typical body archetypes, scientifically known as somatotypes; ectomorphs — the string beans; mesomorphs — the perfect physiques; endomorphs — the plump ones. My body image at the time was that of an endomorph and I knew that I would have been mortified to display my physique to the class.

Both Phillip Valentine Tobias and Paul R Levy were confirmed bachelors, fully dedicating their lives to academics and the university life.

Chapter 7. Examinations in the pre-clinical years

I personally experienced the link between the immune system and neurobiology. This epiphany was the result of being a nasal carrier of the *Staphylococcus* bug, and in the weeks prior to all final examinations I routinely developed a painful boil around the nose. We knew little about the immune system in those days and even less about neurobiology, but there was already a long standing belief that stress and disease were intimately related. I now had good anecdotal "proof".

The practical examination in zoology during the first year was a challenge. We were instructed to dissect some critical parts of a grasshopper, following which we had to disassemble, display and draw the arterial system of a frog. I duly collected my grasshopper from the communal grasshopper box. While pinning it to the cork board it became reanimated, leaping to the floor. I followed it, chasing the grasshopper across the floor of the laboratory on hands and knees. An examiner wisely suggested that I select another specimen. This second one was certifiably dead, and probably had been so for a number years. When I opened it there was nothing inside — a mere dried out husk. Third try was more successful.

The frog dissection did not go well. I plucked an African three- toed frog (*Xenopus laevis*) from the tank, and attempted to dispatch it with the usual pithing procedure. This somewhat resembles the way bull-fighters end the life of the bull by piercing the spinal cord with a long sharp point. It is a tricky maneuver. Eventually my frog stopped protesting and I began the task of revealing its major arteries. Unfortunately I removed one by mistake. Immediately recognizing the error, I set about creating a "fake" vessel by gently teasing the soft tissues with a pair of forceps into something that resembled an artery. With care and patience I actually forged a credible structure. When the examiner stopped by to review my work, he missed the deception and congratulated me for an outstanding dissection. That's when I learned that an ounce of perception is worth a pound of performance.

In addition to gross anatomy, many hours were spent in front of microscopes, peering at slides of various cells and tissues. Known as microscopic anatomy, it was preparation for pathology. Recognizing the abnormal first requires an appreciation of the range of normal. For the end-of-year examination dozens of microscopes were lined up on the laboratory benches, each with a glass slide. Students played musical chairs. Every five minutes a bell sounded and we moved one chair to the left. During the time at the 'scope we had to identify the cell or tissue and answer a number of questions on the examination sheet.

I recall two slides in detail. We all knew that one of the examiners had a bizarre and somewhat sadistic sense of humor. The first problem slide I encountered contained many different tissues all jumbled together. This was not normal, but looked like a tumor known as a teratoma. On the other hand, we were not being tested on pathology. For some reason I took the slide off the microscope's stage and looked at it. The profile of the tissue was perfectly round, a little larger than a nickel. Then the penny dropped — that mixture, with a predominance of muscle, but with fragments of fat, bone, hair, skin, intestine had to be a cross section of a hot dog. And once I saw an insect part, I knew I was correct. The second posed a similar problem of mixed tissues suggesting a more embryonic tumor. Once again I removed the slide and looked at the shape. It was an obvious section of a normal fetal foot. This episode was so influential that for the rest of my professional career I always looked at the slide carefully before putting it on the microscope. And more than once it helped to avoid an embarrassment.

A couple of years later we were all frantically preparing for the practical examination in pathology The buzz round the class was who were going to be the unlucky ones assigned to the external examiner from the University of Cape Town. As there were only a small number of medical schools in South Africa, a collaborative system of sharing examiners had developed over the years. This served a number of useful purposes. It ensured uniform standards between the universities, and neutralized any personal issues between a particular student and a professor. Essentially we were all on a level playing field, or so the theory went. We suspected that is was a ruse to allow faculty to travel and socialize.

There was one legendary professor from Cape Town. Descriptions about his examination technique swirled around the campus leading up to the oral

41

portion of the examination. And he was easy to recognize, we were told, with bright orange hair and bushy ginger eyebrows.

On the morning of the examination we all gathered in the foyer of the pathology museum. The departmental secretary had the class list in front of her on a small table outside the main door. As I approached, she looked up, smiled sweetly, trying to calm our nerves and said, "Ah, Mr. Benjamin, you go to table three." I entered the museum and looked for table three. As my eyes locked onto the number, the table was eclipsed by two huge bushy orange eyebrows. My sweat glands began secreting in earnest and my pulse breached a hundred. After saying good morning, I sat down to face my inquisitors. On the table, in glass or acrylic bottles, were three or four specimens of diseased organs or unidentifiable fragments of presumably human tissue floating in formaldehyde. Professor Becker, the owner of the orange pelage, had a small writing pad on the table in full view of the student, a pencil dangling just above it. He pointed at a specimen — a stag-horn shaped stone inhabiting the middle of a bisected kidney — and asked the first question. I blurted out an answer. His pencil did not move. Next question. This time he drew a long line on the paper. It was abundantly clear that he was beginning to draw a hangman. If he completed the gallows and noose before the end of the examination you already knew your fate — you had failed.

Some suggested that this technique was no more than early training on how to make good decisions under extreme duress. Others termed it torture. It was not explicitly prohibited by the Geneva Convention. Each can decide for themselves the value of such an approach. As I arose to move to the next part of the examination, I was pleased to see that the noose had not been added.

I had dodged yet another bullet on the road to becoming a physician.

Chapter 8. Pathology and vices

Entering an inconspicuous side door at the Johannesburg General Hospital near a loading dock, I joined a group of disconsolate third year medical students at 8 am, all heading to the basement and the ghoul center of the hospital — the autopsy room and theatre. This was the year we were introduced to many of mankind's ills. Anatomy and physiology had introduced us to what is supposedly normal. The third year was devoted to the abnormal — to pathology.

The traditional method of learning this discipline is at the autopsy table. The word itself is quite telling, derived from "to see for oneself."
The technique goes back to the days of the Enlightenment, and perfected by scientists like Rokitansky, who developed the method of removing all the organs with the fewest number of knife strokes. The public's general impression is that an autopsy is performed to determine the cause of death. I was later to learn that it was more useful in determining how the patient lived. It is the ultimate quality assurance mechanism of medical care and its decline in recent decades is to be decried.

Our daily routine was simple. We began each day watching an autopsy — not the easiest fare to wake up to. This was conducted at the Johannesburg General Hospital across the road from the medical school which boasted an autopsy "theatre" accommodating about half the class, although little could be seen from the upper tiers. The back seats were a good place to catch up on sleep. One avoided being in the front rows where one was sure to be questioned. Some of the pathologists caught onto this chicanery and would scan the higher seats to select a victim, who was then invited to describe the findings to the class. Inevitably this metamorphosed into a public humiliation.

Humiliation was a prime motivational technique employed by educators at that time. Facing one's classmates, burbling out some response, only to be met with a sneer and a snide remark from the teacher. It was an awesome tactic. It could only be avoided by hiding or by studying. All this changed in the following decades when students were praised for knowing little, as long as their feelings were acknowledged and their efforts were validated. But these were still the days of high expectations.

The proceedings in the autopsy room were directed by a diener, a kinder word for the assistant ghoul. The diener at the "Gen", Mr Momson, was notorious for his foul language, coarse and crude manner. He was nicknamed "Moofalong Momson" as he hurried us in and out of his autopsy suite. He was despised by all who met him, especially if one happened to cross him. He regarded medical students as the lowest form of life, mere irritants that delayed him finishing his daily duties.

It was then that we discovered another unpleasant fact about life in South Africa at that time, not that we were unaccustomed to unpleasant facts. After all, this was the zenith of the apartheid era. We learned that the non-white students in the class, which included the few Indians and Chinese, were prohibited from watching an autopsy if the corpse was white. The issue seemed to be that the deceased, and perhaps their family, would not take kindly to be seen naked by others who were not members of their approved clan.

General protests against many government policies were beginning in earnest at this time, lead by a remarkable group of women called the Black Sash, an emblem they wore during their silent, non-violent vigils. Bolstered by this, we confronted the authorities and reached a solution that was not perfect, but was perfectly South African — a compromise that allowed all to save face. It mollified our concerns and underscored the absurdity and irrationality of the system. If the patient was white, the diener would remove all the organs and lay them out on the dissection slab and cover the body. Then all of us were permitted to enter the autopsy theatre. So the recently departed would never know that he, or even worse she, had been glimpsed by a non-white. Reminiscing now, one realizes how ridiculous this was. At the time we thought that we had won a great victory against the system, which in fact it was. Such were the vagaries of living with apartheid.

I recall an autopsy conducted by a pathologist affiliated with the Chamber of Mines. Lung diseases are of major concern in the mining industry, and these pathologists probably knew more about silicosis, black lung disease from coal, and asbestosis from the deep gold mines than any others in the world. This particular pathologist was performing an autopsy on an unfortunate who had succumbed to lung cancer, a rising scourge at the time.

Whenever he pontificated over some subtle point of anatomy or pathology, he would rest his lit stogie on the cold marble autopsy bench, then pick it up with his bloody gloved fingers and take a deep draw. "And you do realize, ladies and gentlemen, that tobacco is the obvious cause of most cases of lung cancer. Tobacco smoke contains abundant tars and many other known carcinogens." This was at least two decades before the tobacco companies finally admitted that they knew it all along. For us this was no secret, but being indestructible youth and wanting to emulate our movie heroes, all of whom smoked, we ignored the warning.

Cigarettes were only one of the vices we indulged in. Like most students, alcohol was another. But unlike in the USA at the time, neither marijuana nor psychedelic mushrooms played much part in our chemical recreation. Marijuana, colloquially known as "dagga," was widely available, but the penalties for possession were so stringent that most of us were unwilling to take the risk. Judicial sentences at the time in South Africa included such punishments as "twelve stokes with a heavy cane"; something none of us wished to endure.

Chapter 9. Forensics

Arriving anxious one morning at the Government Laboratories, the forensic pathologist's secretary escorted a small group of us into a cavernous hall. She pointed to one of the many tables that filled the morgue, half of which were occupied by corpses. The one she indicated was presided over by a short stocky man wearing a filthy, blood stained plastic apron. His rubber boots were covered with brown, old caked blood. Smoke curled from a cigar that he had laid on the edge of the concrete slab. His back was towards us. We approached gingerly and then one of us had the temerity to say, "Good morning, Sir. We are the group scheduled for today's case." He spun around and glared. We had interrupted a busy day, and he was in no mood to spend any time teaching medical students. He stared icily at us and said nothing. The victim on the cold slab had succumbed to multiple stab wounds. Such injuries were very common in South Africa, as guns were not widely available, so most disputes or feuds were settled with knives or clubs, the latter under the colloquial name of knobkerrie.

The pathologist picked up a huge knife from the instrument tray, of the type used to slice liver. Think 14-inch chefs knife. He turned to the corpse splayed out on the concrete slab and, in a single stroke, buried it to its hilt in the chest. He pointed at me, gesturing with his fingers to come to the table. "Now describe to your colleagues the difference between a pre-mortem and a post-mortem stab wound." I was speechless for a moment and then muttered a few words, which obviously did not please him. "Have you no eyes? Are you unable to make a simple observation? Can't you think? God, what sort of students are they letting in these days?"

Needless to say this was not a good start to my forensic education, but the graduation requirements were such that we had to attend a minimum number of forensic autopsies, which were assiduously tracked with an attendance record. All of us just met the minimum requirement. Each week we hoped that the case would be a simple clean homicide or suicide; not a burn victim, termed "crispy critters", or a drowning which produced a "purple floating bloater". And then there was always fear of the maggots if a corpse was found many days after death.

Forensics was a long standing tradition in all British inspired medical education. Indeed, forensic pathology was an accepted and important academic discipline. Perhaps it was the Sherlock Holmes effect, but places like Scotland Yard always used the formally trained forensic pathologists from The University of London (Guy's Hospital) for their high profile cases. I was later shocked to discover that such a system did not exist in the USA. The coroner system that had developed in the States is a political amateurish mess, apart from some excellent medical examiners in a few big cities. It dawned on me that if one wanted to dispatch someone and not be caught, the USA was the country for such a deed. We will return to this theme later — not plotting murder, but the sorry condition of forensic pathology.

At this juncture in our training we were far more interested in the living than the dead, and so none looked forward to the weekly trek to the government laboratories for our dose of forensics.

The lectures on the other hand were less intimidating. Some were even interesting. The highlight of the course was the visit from Sir Keith Simpson, perhaps the most famous forensic pathologist in the world at the time. He had written the textbooks on forensic pathology and reportedly had done more autopsies than anyone on earth. Among his more famous cases were the acid bath murders of John Haig, during which he uncovered gallstones and dentures in the fatty sludge in the bath and was able to identify one of the victims. He was even employed by what was the country of Siam (now Thailand) to investigate the death of the king in 1948.

His lecture was riveting. I recall one slide which showed a severed hand brought to him by Scotland Yard. It had been found in a London park. He instantly recognized that it was a prank being played by a group of medical students from one of the local universities. The clue was that a couple of muscles had been carefully dissected. Sir Simpson's autobiography, *Forty Years of Murder*, became a bestseller. Even so, most of us were merely satisfied with passing the forensic examinations with a minimum of work or much investment of time. None of us had any pretensions of going into the field as a career.

Many decades latter, forensics developed a certain cachet, attracting a new generation of Sherlock Holmes wannabes. The field expanded to dental, computer, finance, genocide, toxicology, botany, archeology and many other fields, although traditional medical forensics languished in a backwater despite television programs such as CSI (Crime Scene Investigation), which over romanticized the field. This depiction bears little resemblance to reality, a problem with most reality shows.

In part, the interest in forensic sciences was spawned by the many new opportunities to commit mayhem, and a variety of glitzy new technologies. In the USA, very-few self-respecting pathology residents ever considered a career in forensics. Not only are there no formal training programs, apart from a small number of fellowships, nor any academic recognition, but it was regarded as something that one did if you could not get a real job. In spite of this, some superb forensic pathologists rose to prominence in the USA in medical examiners offices such as LA County, New York, Allegheny County (PA), Dallas County (TX), Dade County (FL), King County (WA) and others.

Despite my disdain for this discipline, two decades later I was deputized to be a medical examiner. But this tale will have to wait.

Chapter 10. The Conference

During the 1960s there were only five medical schools in South Africa. A couple have been added since. As was common at that time the schools were segregated by language and race. Two of them used Afrikaans, while three taught in English, but one of the latter, in Durban, was reserved for the "non-Europeans." This was a very nebulous designation, but included the entire black population. Other ethnic groups such as East Indians, Coloreds (mixed race), and Chinese occupied an uneasy place, with some being admitted to the "white-only" schools. The English-speaking schools all shared an affinity, not the least of which was a general rejection of the ruling government's apartheid policies, and an antipathy to having to speaking Afrikaans to patients of that ilk.

This put us at serious odds with the authorities. And there was lots to fight against, some serious, some trivial. On the trivial end of this spectrum was a law that prohibited whites from serving alcohol in any of its varieties to blacks. At the other end was the strict prohibition of any physical contact between the so-called "races," enshrined in a law known as the Immorality Act. This was much more serious, with the potential for years in prison. As students, we had to find ways to navigate and circumvent all these laws.

The three English-speaking medical schools had an annual conference tradition hosted on a rotating basis at one of the campuses. These were semi-formal affairs featuring scientific sessions at which students presented their research, athletic events, and lots of socializing. The latter featured considerable quantities of alcohol, music, dancing and extensive fraternizing. The local nursing schools were also willing participants in these events. To obviate the problem of serving alcohol, we devised a simple expedient. No matter where the conference was held, we always declared the Durban school as the official host. As it was designated as being black, there was no problem serving alcohol to everyone. The authorities probably detected this deception, but turned a blind eye.

Fraternizing was far more problematic. At one of the conferences held in CapeTown, I met and developed a relationship with an exquisite East Indian Sikh nurse from Durban. We corresponded over the year and planned to meet up again at the next conference which happened to be in Durban. She attended my boring presentation on aspirin poisoning in children. I offered her a ride back to her home on the outskirts of town. As we drove out of the parking lot an unmarked police cruiser began following us, at a discrete, but warning distance. We made sure to keep ample space between the two of us, even though in those days the car seats were like sofas, as bucket seats were reserved for sport cars. The police vehicle accompanied us for over twenty miles until we arrived at her home where she alighted and casually waved goodbye to both me and our personal police escort. They followed me back to medical school. Probably added another line in my official dossier.

That was the last time I ever saw her. There are some special people one never forgets.

Chapter 11. Head games

"Gentlemen, I have arranged a special treat for you today. You are going to interview one of our newest and most fascinating patients. Take a seat and I will bring her to you."

We were on a field trip to Sterkfontein Psychiatric Hospital, a state-run institution located in Krugersdorp adjacent to Johannesburg. It was also where accused murderers were committed for psychiatric examination prior to trial. In the center of the sprawling campus was a high security prison to which they were consigned. These were euphemistically known as the forensic wards, and this is where the interview was to be conducted.

The psychiatrist then gave us a brief brief about the upcoming interview. A colleague and myself were about to meet an actress who had recently dispatched three lives. She had killed her husband, then axed her lover to death on the following day. After being committed for psychiatric evaluation, she entered into a suicide pact with one of her nurses. The plan they hatched to use the carbon monoxide from the nurse's car as their mode of exit. After the exhaust was hooked up, the murderess bumped her door open, managing to breathe enough fresh air, while her nursing companion turned rosy red and succumbed to the fumes in the seat beside her.

The two of us were ushered into a small room, waiting anxiously for what was about to transpire. The staff psychiatrist and an extremely attractive young woman entered together. He introduced us and then immediately left, locking the door from the outside. This was disconcerting. But the next hour was remarkable. In another setting she would have been the life and soul of any party — witty, engaging, amusing and totally disconnected from reality. "Well," she said, about the events of the past month, "those are just the sort of things that sometimes happen in life. I think that I would still like to become a missionary nurse." I do not know what ultimately became of her. I don't even know if she was declared mentally fit to stand trial. I doubt she married again.

Of course, she might have been deceiving us all the time. It was around this period that an iconic study was reported in the psychiatric literature. Completely normal people were secretly admitted to a mental hospital for evaluation. After a relatively brief time the only people who recognized that they were entirely normal were the inmates. The medical and nursing staff all thought they were nuts with a variety of different psychiatric disorders. A classic example of expectations eclipsing reality.

I did not take readily to psychiatry. In addition to the standard boring lectures, we were taken to a variety of mental institutions, many of which recalled the awful scenes at Bedlam in the eighteenth century. Even though I regard myself as reasonably empathetic, I am uncomfortable around certifiably crazy folk, or those with serious mental retardation. The classification system for the latter was still rather primitive at the time — morons, imbeciles, idiots — based on some specious measurements of intelligence. Even so there was little doubt that their mental aptitudes were clearly below par.

There were not yet ICD codes with which to pigeonhole a behavior we did not understand or claim reimbursement for our treatments. In addition to a few drugs which seriously impaired any ability to function, the occasional lobotomy was still being performed, and we watched with horror as electroconvulsive therapy was administered to particularly fractious patients. While this was bad enough for the white patients, at least they received a general anesthetic prior to having the electrodes discharge large amounts of energy through their brain. Black patients were not so fortunate, although they did become unconscious within milliseconds of the power being switched on, and the beginning of violent convulsions.

We saw entire wards filled with patients with severe hydrocephalus, massive swollen heads looking like aliens from another planet. Models for ET. Many wards had polished concrete floors with a single drain in the middle and simple iron cots so that it could be hosed down a couple times a day. This was the stuff of nightmares — humanoids eking out a survival of sorts. My sympathies were also with the caregivers. This experience also raised deep philosophical questions about society and humanity; questions that probably have no satisfactory answers.

Part of the final examination in psychiatry was conducted at this same facility, although not in the maximum security area. A large hall was filled with tables, each with two chairs. Patients were brought in and seated opposite a medical student. We were given three hours to interview our patient and write a report including an assessment, diagnosis and treatment plan. I had a run-of the mill schizophrenic. The patient at the table next to me said a few words to the examining student, and then spent the rest of the time crawling around the room picking up cigarette butts, smoking and drooling. The medical student spent the three hours busily writing. After the examination ended I asked him what had happened. "Oh," he said, "it was really easy. My patient sat down and announced that he had spoken to God when he awoke that morning. God said that medical students were coming to examine him. And then God said, "There is no need to waste your time with the student. Just tell him to speak directly to me. I will tell him all that he needs to know."

That was all I needed to know that psychiatry was not in my future.

Chapter 12 - The 'Viva'; Clinical Examination Time

Examination time, as it is for all students everywhere regardless of discipline, was especially stressful. Preparing for the clinical examinations became high art. One of the techniques was to go to Baragwanath Hospital on a weekend and ask a registrar for a list of patients whose pathology we thought might be important to know. "Go to beds 14, 18, 21, 13 in ward 18 B to examine patients with mitral stenosis." In an hour we probably saw and examined more patients with this disorder than the average overseas medical student would have seen during their entire training. After examining a patient we would present the case to a colleague, as if they were the examiner. This was serious role-playing and excellent preparation for the real thing.

During the clinical years the most important part of the examinations was devoted to live, hands-on, oral examinations, known as "vivas." The written portions of the exams were generally essay style, often with a choice to answer three out of five possible topics. Multiple choice examinations of the style that became popular in later years were unheard of. These have also been termed multiple guess.

The essay selection was never straightforward. Questions like "discuss the embryology and anatomy of the bare area of the spleen"; or "evaluate the molecular structure of water in relation to human biology"; or "discuss the pathophysiologic changes in metabolism following major trauma."

A number of what might have been regarded as semi-professional patients were employed every year for examinations. They might have a unique or a rare disease, an interesting physical finding or could otherwise test a student's ability to take a good history or notice a subtle physical sign. Some were skilled at deception, others were quite helpful if they felt sorry for a hapless student.

We evaluated various techniques to be successful at the vivas. A standard method was to keep talking as long as possible, giving the examiners less time to ask questions. The examiners themselves seemed to follow two major tactics. The first method was to go deep — to keep asking more and more penetrating questions on the same topic until the student said, "I don't know the answer to that, sir." The second technique was to go broad. As soon as they sensed that a student knew an acceptable answer, they would ask another question on another topic until the student said, "I don't know." Regardless of the method, one always left the examination only remembering the times that one said "I don't know." And that convinced one of failure, conveniently forgetting the 98 questions one had answered correctly.

I will never forget three particular final examinations. The first was an obstetrics viva. A plaster cast of a pelvis, a plastic baby doll, two examiners and a set of forceps greeted me in the examination room. "Mr. Benjamin, please place the infant with the head in a left occiput anterior position and perform a low outlet forceps delivery." I dutifully positioned the baby with the head in the appropriate position. Despite having done a score of forceps deliveries, I picked up the wrong blade and inserted it. Immediately I recognized the error and began to giggle. The reason for the laugh was I recalled the story recounted in *Doctor in the House*, in which a medical student was confronted with just this situation. The "Doctor" series of books, popular in the

1960s, was written by a London surgeon/ anesthesiologist (Richard Gordon) and became a memorable TV show on BBC. Although fictitious, the antics of a group of medical students at St. Swithins were the stuff of legend. Legends we were actively living out.

In the story, the medical student put the forceps blades in correctly and began to pull. When the head didn't move he placed one foot against the table and really tugged. When that failed, he put both feet against the bed and yanked. The pelvis flew over his head, the baby doll landed in a corner and the forceps blades lay on the floor. One examiner picked up a blade, handed it back to the student and said, "Now, Mr. Smith, why don't you take this and hit the father over the head and then you would have killed the whole family." This image flooded back to me, and for an instant I thought I was in a comic living nightmare.

"Mr. Benjamin, is there a reason for your mirth? Will you share what is so amusing?" I got myself back under control and said, "Sir, do you mind if I start again from the beginning?"

The second episode was during a gynecological examination. I don't' recall the specifics of the patient or her problems — most likely uterine fibroids, a common and readily diagnosable condition. I completed the examination, discussed the findings and management. The examiners asked repeatedly if I had missed anything or if there was anything else to report. I was vehement that my examination and assessment was complete. Until I walked out of the door. Then I remembered that I had failed to do a rectal examination. This despite a medical aphorism that I had heard many times: "If you don't put your finger in it, you put your foot in it."

The third event was during a oral examination in general medicine. The patient had a condition for which aspirin was the appropriate first agent to use to control the symptoms. By chance, during a rotation at children's hospital, I had admitted a child with salicylate poisoning. I became interested in the topic, reviewed all the cases in the poison center's records from the prior decades, and prepared a paper for publication, as well as presenting the findings at a student conference. At the end of this I probably knew as much about aspirin and its side effects as anyone at that time.

At the conclusion of my presentation of the case and diagnosis, I began pontificating about the treatment. "Salicylates would be my first choice of medication," I said, "but there are possible side effects." One of the examiners then said, "Oh, would you like to inform us what those might be?" That was the cue I needed to launch into a fifteen-minute exposition. I hardly took a breath during this time so that they would not be able to interrupt or stop me. It was the only question they asked.

Success at examinations is a strange, almost intuitive skill. Some of my colleagues, far more knowledgeable than I, often performed poorly. Others, who would become much better physicians, did not demonstrate their abilities during these examinations. I was very fortunate. I fell into the category of a good exam taker. This always made me feel slightly guilty. It was fascinating how we all knew who the best students were. Asking the class to rank students would be more effective than any external grading system. Of course, this was not the main reason for examinations. The fundamental reason was to ensure that we knew enough to be safe physicians. I recall the foreword of an anesthesiology textbook for medical students that stated this explicitly: "If you can't be good, at least be safe." Sage advice.

One examination still gives me nightmares. During our senior year we were invited to sit for the examination that would permit us to enter the United States. Even though some in the class had no intention of emigrating, it was regarded as an insurance policy, so almost everyone participated. It was administered by an American consular representative under the auspices of the Educational Council For Foreign Medical Graduates (ECFMG) and held in a large hall in downtown Johannesburg.

There were two components. The initial portion was a test of our medical knowledge, conducted with a multiple choice format, the first time any of us had seen this method. I believe the average score in our class was 95%. So that was the easy part. The second portion was a test of spoken English. I had to deal with two issues, sitting in the back row. The hall abutted a major bus route through the city. The noise of the buses driving by made it hard to hear anything. The consul, recognizing this problem, paused with his question, but began talking just as the bus reached me. The second problem was that he was from Georgia, with a deep southern accent. Even though we had been raised on American movies, this was like nothing we had heard before. He asked, "What is a *heeeeal*?" I looked at the answer sheet and had to select from a. the bottom of a shoe, b. a small mountain, c. a cure d. none of the above.

By the end of the examination I was convinced that I had failed American English.

13. The Midwife

In South Africa the overwhelming majority of deliveries were performed by midwives, a secret sect whose second mission, after helping women through the difficulties of childbirth, was the humiliation of medical students. They were brilliant at both. Unlike the USA where general hospitals are expected to cover the medical waterfront, South Africa, mimicking the UK after which the system was modeled, had any number of specialty hospitals. This included Fever Hospital, for infectious communicable diseases, an eye hospital, a children's hospital, and naturally, a maternity hospital. If one didn't deliver at home this is where babies entered the world. The Queen Victoria Maternity Hospital was just over the hill from medical school and the Johannesburg General Hospital. It was opposite The Fort, a structure dating back before the Boer War, which became a jail and is currently a museum. The complex of buildings is now called Constitution Hill, which is perhaps more of a hope than a reality.

The "Vic" was where white "European" women delivered their babies and where we were sent for our first tour of obstetrics. There was not a

71

designated maternity hospital for the black population in central Johannesburg, so prospective mothers had to travel to outlying hospitals.

It was also one of the first living-in experiences for us as students. Simple bedrooms arranged along a single corridor were dedicated for us while we waited to be summoned for a delivery, or to recover from being semi-conscious and exhausted. The most prominent structure in the room, aside from a single narrow bed, was a large bell on the wall — the signal to immediately go to the delivery area.

As students, we were under the strict supervision of the midwives and were required to follow their instructions to the letter. They did have a lot of letters. A delivery was a carefully choreographed affair in which ritual and tradition played large roles. A mother was required to lie on her back and the attendant — either student or midwife, was always on the patient's right side. Too bad if one was left handed. Later we learned that many African woman much preferred to squat during delivery, a more effective method of giving birth. It creates a better anatomical position, and gravity is an added benefit. It suited all the participants except the midwives. White women were permitted to walk around prior to delivery, but once in labor it was back to their backs.

The birth of a human infant is incontrovertible evidence against "Intelligent Design." No sentient force would ever devise such an awkward and dangerous process. The problem that evolution has created is two fold. Because we are bipedal and spend most of our time upright, the pelvis, through which the baby is expected to pass, has changed shape. Compounding the problem, our heads are too big because of a large brain. In order for the head to pass through the birth canal we are born before we are really ripe enough for the world. Most other mammals deliver offspring that are fully prepared to enter the outside world — they can see, walk, hear and even run after a day or two. Humans, on the other hand, are perfectly helpless for many months. The combination of an oversized head and a narrow birth canal is potentially fraught with problems. Midwives were experts at mitigating most of these difficulties, and when they were not able to, an obstetrician was nearby with an array of medieval instruments or a scalpel. But unlike the USA, where over 35% of all deliveries are by cesarean section, the rate in South Africa was below 5%. Despite this, most of us turned out okay.

The birthing process is a really messy business, not for the faint-hearted. The old Latin aphorism, ascribed to St Augustine, describes it well — *"Inter faeces et urinam nascimur."* (We are born between shit and piss) To that needs to be added amniotic fluid, which has a distinctive bouquet, and blood and mucus.

Part of the ritual was to assign a medical student to a fully gravid woman from the moment she was admitted until some hours after delivery. This meant sitting at the bedside for many hours and on a few occasions, even days. We always hoped that the admitting doctor or midwife had adequately assessed the stage of labor or, even better, that the mother had already given birth to a passel of kids, as their time in labor was generally much briefer.

Everyone knew that the system was rigged against medical students. It was at the discretion of the head nurse to allot cases to either a student nurse or a medical student, rather than on a strict rotational basis. Usually the "multips" were entrusted to the midwifery students. Such multips (from "multiparous") generally had short labors. Primiparous women ("primips") on the other hand were unpredictable, often in labor for many hours. Certain ethnic groups had determined that screaming during delivery was not just expected, it was important for the soul of the baby. We were never assigned to "elderly primips" as they were regarded as high risk and needed more expert care than a mere medical student could provide. This moniker was applied to any woman over 35 years having her first pregnancy. I recall the chagrin my wife expressed when she saw "elderly primip" on her own chart, even though she had not attained the official age.

Sitting with a woman through hours of early labor was tedious and boring. We timed contractions, documenting their duration and strength. We recorded the baby's heart rate and rhythm with a fetoscope — essentially a modified stethoscope. We massaged backs. And we waited. Most fathers on the other hand waited in the waiting room and could smoke, drink coffee and socialize. Every now and then we would assess the state of the cervix, the position of the skull and how labor was progressing. And, if all went well, we handled the delivery.

But that was not the end. The placenta had to be carefully examined to ensure that it was completely intact with no missing bits and pieces. The student was then tasked with taking the newborn to nursery, cleaning off the bodily fluids, waiting for the baby's clinical condition and temperature to stabilize, bathing the infant until its skin was bright and shiny, and then returning the newborn to the mother with a smile. After eighteen hours of a labor and delivery, all we wanted was sleep.

A colleague came up with a brilliant plot to avoid these post-delivery responsibilities. After his second delivery he waited until the head nurse — the matron — was patrolling the nursery. He entered, filled the tub with boiling water and asked which bassinet baby Smith was in. He grabbed the infant by the feet, and casually walked over to the tub as if he was going to dunk the newborn head first into the steaming cauldron. Horror swept through the nursery. The Matron yelled, "Mr. X, you are not permitted to ever step foot in this nursery again."

Problem solved.

Chapter 14. Party time at the 'Vic.'

Obstetric training at the Queen Victoria Maternity Hospital — the "Vic", was one of many enjoyable living-in training experiences. Admittedly there were times after monitoring a very long labor and delivery that one was exhausted, but, between these times, there was ample time to relax and play. Staff tennis courts were available to us, as well as a welcome bed in the medical student quarters. The food in the staff dining room was passable.

Young student midwives were also trained at the "Vic." Opportunities for fraternizing were endless, despite the explicit prohibition of nursing students and medical students ever occupying the same corridor, let alone the same bedroom. While we were not required to sign a legal injunction, there was little doubt that any breach of this unwritten policy would result in serious consequences.

Most of us were still young and in the latter stages of the post-adolescent hormone storm. There was an air of playfulness, and we indulged in a variety of childish shenanigans. Nurses delighted in replacing the milk in the refrigerator that we used for tea or coffee with expressed breast milk, just to watch our reaction when we tasted the slightly different sweetness. A favorite betting game was to fill rubber surgical gloves with water and race them down the stairs — years before the slinky became a popular children's toy.

One week we decided to have a joint party with the student midwives and managed to convince a local brewery to donate beer to the cause. I drove over to the brewery with a friend. On arrival at the loading dock, I was asked how many cases I needed. "As much as you can give. We plan to christen the whole hospital, " I responded. This left no room in the car for my companion who had to take a bus back to the "Vic." The car was so laden, I was concerned for the springs. The next problem was smuggling the beer into the hospital unseen. I parked the car near the admissions area and wheeled out a patient trolley, loaded it up, covering the evidence with a couple of sheets.

The next day, while doing a pelvic examination with the chief obstetrician, he casually said to me, "I believe you brought some beer into the hospital yesterday, Benjamin." Fearing the worst, I knew that I had to admit. He turned to me and gruffly said, "So why the hell have I not been invited to the party?" He received an instant invitation.

It was after he left that things got really dicey. The party was a great success, and late at night we attempted to smuggle a couple of nurses into the medical student corridor. Just when we thought we had succeeded, the elevator door at the end of the hall opened, and there stood the night-matron.

The next day a couple of us were summoned for an interrogation with the chief obstetrician and head matron. Once again I imagined that my medical school days were over. We were reprimanded with a few smiles that "boys will be boys." The nursing students were expelled because they "should have known better."

Fifty years later I still regret this event. They would have become excellent midwives. This epitomized the double standards present then and which remain largely intact today.

Chapter 15. High on obstetrics

The second stint in obstetrics was a month-long rotation at Edendale hospital in Natal (now Kwa-Zulu, Natal) near Pietermaritzburg, on the way to Durban. This hospital served the rural black population. Of the 900 beds, a substantial fraction were devoted to obstetrics. By this stage of our training we were seasoned veterans in obstetrics, having performed far more deliveries than most medical students in other countries. But Edendale was the chance to get some serious experience. The requirements were to perform a large number of normal deliveries, fifty I recall; low and mid outlet forceps, vacuum extraction (Ventouse), some twin deliveries, breach and footling deliveries, and be first assistant at a number of cesarean sections. We were also expected to participate in the management of the usual obstetric emergencies such as prolapsed cord, a transverse lie, massive hemorrhage, severe eclampsia and all the rest.

In the week prior to this road trip, a pharmaceutical representative (aka salesman or drug pusher) had stopped by the ward during the morning tea break. In his bag of free samples was a new agent for weight loss. His sales pitch was impressive — guaranteed appetite suppressant, few side effects, etc. I imagined that I was becoming a little plump as I loved food. I took a few bottles of his latest nostrum to try. Almost immediately I lost any desire to eat. I also couldn't sleep and was almost manic. By the time we got to Edendale I decided that since I couldn't sleep I would complete all my deliveries as rapidly as possible and then have time to play on the beaches of Durban or in the Drakensberg Mountains.

Unlike our experience at the Queen Victoria Maternity Hospital where we had to be present at a delivery from start to finish, at Edendale we were only required to perform the delivery. Perform is not quite the right word. The mothers performed, we merely stood by, cheered them on, occasionally provided some assistance, sutured any tears, helped name the baby, and then moved on to the next delivery. In three or four days I had completed my requirement — fifty normal deliveries. I then requested that I only be summoned for the complicated cases.

I had lost about ten pounds. But something was seriously wrong. I then learned that this weight loss agent was no more than a variant of dexedrine, an amphetamine, and despite the drug representative's pitch, it had all the side effects and more. Realizing the addictive potential, I stopped the pills, which is much easier said than done. I still have great sympathy for those in the profession and our patients who become victims of the pharmaceutical industry. I was lucky. There is nothing that the industry can do that will bring back my trust. If anything, it has gotten progressively worse, which turned me into a lifelong therapeutic nihilist.

Having completed all the obstetrics that was expected, we had abundant time to play. Durban was only a hour or so away, Gray's Hospital in Pietermaritzburg had a large nursing school, most of the students being young nubile women, and the resorts and parks of the Drakensberg Mountains were within easy driving distance. From what I recall it was a memorable month. I even considered obstetrics as a specialty for my future. It was largely caring for young, reasonably healthy patients and the outcomes, for the most part were happy events. It did have its messy moments, but not as noxious as some other specialties such as pathology. Patients were generally appreciative. Some even wanted to name their infant after the person who performed the delivery. One of my colleagues was chagrined when the birth mother asked for his name and then said, "What a pity it's not a nice name."

One of the more interesting rotations in our senior year was at the clinic in Alexandra Township on the north side of Johannesburg. This sprawling ghetto on the banks of the Jukskei River consisted of small huts, shacks and houses, unpaved roads, coal fires and shebeens (speakeasies), housing up to 50,000 people, including at one time residents such as Nelson Mandela, Hugh Masekela, and in later years Trevor Noah. There was even a plan to demolish it and replace the homes with single-sex hostels, similar to the accommodation on the goldmines for the itinerant black labor force. This never occurred.

The university helped run a clinic which provided all the health care for the entire population, although the local *sangomas* and *inyanga* (medicine men/women and herbalists) probably cared for a lot more patients than the clinic. During the day a small medical staff was on site, but after dark, the clinic was turned over to a cadre of outstanding nurses, senior medical students and an ambulance driver.

We handled every imaginable emergency, from stab wounds to severely dehydrated infants, and everything in between. One evening a young pregnant women arrived soon after her waters broke with the umbilical cord prolapsed. Normally, this is fatal for the infant unless the baby can be extracted as soon as possible. Fortunately, the one and only ambulance was available, and I was delegated to hold the cord back in place while we drove to the nearest hospital about thirty minutes away. The mother was placed with her head down on her elbows, and her butt in the air with me sitting behind her, holding everything in. Every second I could feel the cord pulsate, hoping that it wouldn't quit before we arrived. A cesarean section was performed within minutes of our arrival. A happy outcome.

Thus ended my obstetrical career. Always good to end on a natural high.

Chapter 16. Leprosy

One of the many strengths of our education during the 1960s was its breadth. Topics barely mentioned in the today's medical school curriculum or which are optional electives, were absolute requirements for us. There were no optional courses — it was all or nothing. We received superb instruction on nutrition, a subject woefully lacking in today's training. It still informs my daily skepticism about the food industry and its marketing. Another topic was public health, appropriately labeled Preventative and Social Medicine. We were dragged to see water purification plants, sewage treatment facilities, and trash disposal. It covered topics such as poverty, causes of human, personal and social disorganization, and medico-social legislation. It also focused on social and industrial diseases including TB, typhus, venereal disease (now under the rubric of sexually transmitted diseases with the acronym of STDs), malaria — which by then had been eradicated in South Africa — and leprosy.

There was one remaining hospital catering to the few remaining lepers. These poor souls had been permanently scarred and disfigured by this disease before adequate treatment became available, so the hospital was more of a sanitarium where they could safely and securely live out the remainder of their lives. One of the public health field trips was to this facility.

We were seated in a stifling hot conference room. Air conditioning was not a luxury in most buildings around Johannesburg, and certainly not one run by the provincial government. Public budgets for health care were not generous. Curtain screens separated medical students from inmates. The medical director called out a name, and the patient went to the front of the room to proudly display his or her lesions. They had done this for so many years that they knew the routine. It was probably a welcome break from the tedium of institutional life. My seat happened to abut the curtain. Every now and then a patient would whisper to me requesting a cigarette. In the background I could also hear a radio owned by one of the patients.

Midway through the afternoon a hand, missing a couple of fingers, was thrust between the curtains directly in front of my face. A small folded piece of paper was wedged between two gnarled stumps. I thought that it was another request for a smoke. I gingerly took the note and opened it. Scrawled in pencil was, *"President Verwoed has just been stabbed to death in parliament."* There was no more surrealistic way to have received this news.

I loved the concept of public health — the idea that a relatively small investment in rather simple methods could have such a huge impact on the health of large populations. It was a blend of science, medicine, economics, policy and politics. It also became apparent that the substantial increase in human longevity, as well as general well being, was the result of basic, common sense and well established public health measures — vaccines, clean water, fresh air, and was not a result to the latest discovery or new technology or building a new hospital. But this is not the stuff that makes headlines.

It is what stimulated my interest in international health, a passion I was fortunately able to pursue later in my career.

Chapter 17. The Firm

Entering the clinical years the class was divided into what were known as "firms" — small groups of medical students who were scheduled for the same rotations, and who attended seminars together. They were like temporary micro-fraternities. Creating these firms was similar to teenage dating or watching puppies sniff around as they assess possible friends. It was important that there was some compatibility and cohesion in the group. Our firm was a rather eclectic assortment of characters, spanning the spectrum from moderately lazy to intense — a nice balance.

Our firm designed a necktie featuring a U-shaped structure reminiscent of a uterus in which was the snake of Asclepius — the classical symbol of healing and medicine. The latter also represented the latest technology in birth control — the Lippies loop, a plastic coil intended to prevent implantation of a fertilized ovum. We thought the design brilliant. No one else had a clue what it signified. We also hoped that it would be a talisman against an unexpected pregnancy.

Each firm had a different personality and vibe depending on its constituents, much like any fraternity or sorority. Most of us lived at home with our parents. Even though medical school was essentially free, many of us looked for small opportunities to supplement our finances to reduce any burden on our family. This varied from being clerks for bookmakers at the horse-races, providing bar service at major cricket or rugby venues, to waiting tables at local restaurants. Perhaps my most unique gig was appearing as an extra in an American movie. The long evening on the set netted me a free dinner and a check for one rand, less ten cents for tax.

One of our firm's members was particularly entrepreneurial. He was more independent than the rest of us, having his own flat. However, this created additional financial strain so that he had a variety of extracurricular jobs to fund his lifestyle. To save even further, he brewed his own alcohol, using mashed up whole pineapples — a very inexpensive fruit — some sugar and yeast. These were packed into mason jars and allowed to ferment.

The resulting alcohol was particularly nasty, but managed to lubricate a number of firm parties —

affairs generally involving medical and nursing students, to which our regular girlfriends preferred not to attend. The downside to this home-brew, other than the taste and terrible hangover, was that some of the mason jars occasionally exploded. To avert catastrophic flooding, they were stored in the bath-tub prior to consumption.

His most creative enterprise was developing a topical application to delay premature ejaculation. This was a simple brew of a local anesthetic, generously provided by a clinic or ward, mixed with KY Jelly. It evidently earned a very devoted following from the staff at one of the restaurants where he moonlighted.

I was once employed by the marketing arm of a pharmaceutical company to conduct interviews with physicians about their use of antibiotics. An elaborate cocktail party was set up behind a one-way mirror with microphones hidden in the decorations. Behind the mirror were the marketing executives. My role was to act as a facilitator and engage the participants in discussion. After a couple of single malt whiskeys or good gins, they would freely discuss when, why and how they used certain medications. Despite being told upfront that they were being observed and recorded, their inhibitions rapidly diminished after the second cocktail. For me it was easy money and very good appetizers.

While all this may sound like fun and games, the final outcome of this group of students was quite remarkable - two pediatric pathologists, a hematologist/blood banker, a plastic surgeon, an ENT surgeon, a pulmonologist, rheumatologist, two neurologists; many with national and/or international reputations and impressive academic careers. And on the side some became notable sculptors and artists.

Perhaps most telling was that eight of the ten left South Africa after their exceptional training — a loss to their home country, but benefitting any number of countries abroad, especially the United States of America and Australia.

Chapter 18. Hypochondriasis

Long before herpes virus, human papilloma virus, chlamydia, HIV and other scourges of promiscuity became commonplace, two old-fashioned diseases, gonorrhea and syphilis were still prevalent, especially in the black population. This was in-spite of the success of antibiotics as standard treatment, a testament to the relative lack of readily available health care for this population. Fortunately the most awful manifestations of syphilis, such as the congenital form in newborns or the madness of tertiary syphilis, were in decline due to therapy.

We were required to attend a monthly venereal disease clinic. This was near the top of our most disliked activities. We stood around the examination table, taking care not to touch anything. At the time someone posted a sign in a toilet stall that warned, "it doesn't' matter if you don't sit down. Spirochetes can jump nine inches." In a few hours we saw ulcers and rashes of various and sundry sizes and colors, and listened to the complaints of burning while urinating, discharges and other miserable symptoms.

During this time I developed a widespread rash, especially on my trunk. It consisted of vaguely copper colored, non-itchy patches. I immediately diagnosed myself as having secondary syphilis. I made an appointment with a dermatologist who was one of the consultants on the medical school faculty. He dutifully took a brief history, learned that I was a medical student and then asked me pull up my shirt. He peered closely at my skin through the bottom of his dermatologist's half-glasses. Then he said, "I don't think that I want to touch you. Do you mind if my partner takes a look at this. And you are a medical student, correct?" By this stage I was a basket case. His partner came in, took a close look and then both began to laugh. "You thought that you had syphilis, didn't you young man?" "What you really have is a completely benign disease called pityriasis rosea. There is a large characteristic 'herald' patch on your back that you can't see. It will all be gone in a couple of weeks." This was the first of a number of fatal diseases that I contracted during my years in medicine. Amazingly I survived them all, albeit with some anxious moments. Hypochondriasis is an occupational hazard, but one seldom discussed or admitted by physicians.

In bygone days it was said that if you knew syphilis you knew medicine. It had protean manifestations, affecting many organs in so many ways, at so many times during its long course. I once owned a large five volume set of antiquarian books entitled *A System of Syphilis*. During our era the same could have been said about tuberculosis. In many situations, especially patients living in rural areas, the first, second and third possibilities for their symptoms was TB. It was still so prevalent that medical students were first tested for TB, and those few of us that were negative were given a vaccination known as BCG, named after the scientist who developed the strain of bacteria for the vaccine (Bacillus Calmette–Guérin). This proved to be a problem after I moved to the USA as all the hospitals required TB testing for the staff. And each year I would have to argue with the occupational nurse that I would be positive because of the vaccine I had received as a student and that the test was a waste of time. But bureaucracy being what it is, the nurse was mandated to check off the little boxes to prove to the powers that she had satisfied the rules. Inevitably there was a new nurse every year.

This was an example of reverse hypochondriasis — me having to convince others that I did not have disease they suspected I had.

19. The Placebo

At Alexandra Clinic, in a black township on the northern edge of white Johannesburg, we began noticing young males arriving after work in the early evenings with vague complaints directed to areas below the belt. It soon became apparent that there were two probable diagnoses — gonorrhea or what they considered impotence. Such erectile dysfunction was clearly in the eye of the beholder, as these were young, healthy virile men for whom any decrease in sexual prowess and performance was a personal concern.

Many cultures have developed ways of dealing with the problem of diminished male performance, employing everything from magic to even more magic. Dozens of herbs, spices, minerals, fragments of animal parts, insects and various incantations have been tried. Even eating stinkhorn mushrooms, which are penile in appearance, require considerable fortitude for consumption. But if one can stomach durian, the foul smelling, although delicious tropical fruit, anything is possible. The little caterpillar fungus from the Tibetan highlands, *Orphicordyceps sinensis* is favored by the colossally rich Chinese, as it more costly than gold and equally ineffective. The issue is so troublesome and potentially lucrative that it enticed pharmaceutical companies to spend billions of dollars to come up with a little blue pill. But that discovery was still years away.

We decided to run a small experiment at the clinic. This was done without sanction from above and long before Institutional Review Boards had to bless any form of medical research. We opted for two types of treatment — conventional Western style psychotherapy or a placebo. In other words we would either have a long discussion about the problem and how it might be mitigated — stress reduction, no alcohol, no dagga (marijuana) — or get a an intradermal injection of sterile water. This was the proverbial dose of a sugar pill, except this water injection was painful.

I was on duty when our first experimental subject arrived. I randomly pulled a treatment card from the file. *Injection.* I approached the patient and said, "This is going to sting, but it will make you much better. Big and strong." He gritted his teeth as I gave the injection. The next evening he returned to the clinic looking for the same doctor who gave him the injection. With him were six friends all wanting the same treatment. Our trial was doomed to fail as the word was out on the street.

A pity we were not in today's environment of the Internet, flim-flam, snake-oil and rampant charlatinism. One could make a fortune with this "muti" (aka medicine). Much like homeopathy.

————————————————

One patient forever changed the way I viewed medicine and healing. He was referred to us from a rural mission hospital. The number of indigenous languages in South Africa made history taking a challenge, sometimes requiring at least two translators. Most of the nurses were reasonably fluent in English, Afrikaans, Xhosa, Zulu and fanagalo (fanakalo). The latter was a mishmash of multiple languages devised on the goldmines for simple communication. Based largely on Zulu, fanagalo was the lingua franca of the mining industry. The word itself means do "like this," the instruction to mimic what the supervisor was doing. There are eleven official languages in South Africa and any number of regional dialects and variations, so at times things got lost in translation. Some nurses did considerable editorializing, telling us what they thought we wanted to hear.

This particular patient arrived arrived on a Thursday with a confusing story about an argument he had had with a neighbor. His antagonist went to the local witchdoctor, who put a curse on the patient. He was told that he was going to die and that the only thing that could save him was an operation in a white man's hospital. He had arrived for his operation. Physically he looked awful and he was admitted to our ward.

There was nothing on the physical examination to account for his condition, and a few simple laboratory tests and X-rays were all normal. I presented the case on ward-rounds the next day. Dr. Seftel instructed, "Benjamin, book the operating room for Monday morning. We will open his belly, suture him back up and he will be fine. I have seen this before and these patients will die."

By Saturday he looked even worse. He had lost more weight in spite of eating, and was getting weaker. On Sunday the registrar called me. "Come over to the ward," he said, "I have an idea." We told the patient that his body was filled with demons and we were going to burn them out of him. To prove it, I took five ccl of his blood and mixed it with hydrogen peroxide. Huge pink bubbles frothed out of the test tube. His eyes widened in horror. "See," we said, "that is what we going to get rid of." We then gave him a large dose of intravenous nicotinic acid (Vitamin B3 or niacin). Given this way it causes immediate flushing and a sensation of heat because of the vasodilatation of vessels in the skin. He lay there "on-fire" for about an hour before we returned. "We need to make sure that there is nothing left behind." Once again I drew some blood, this time mixing it with water. No bubbles or effervescence. In the evening the nurse called me to say that the patient was looking much better. We cancelled the operating room, and discharged him after a couple of days. At follow-up clinic three months later, he was fine. We had finally beaten Seftel at his own game — understanding and appreciating culture and one's personal beliefs about illness.

The placebo effect is one of the most powerful instruments in a physicians black bag. We were instructed to use it wisely. It could be as powerful as the other mainstay of healing — "the tincture of time."

Chapter 20. Physical diagnosis

The art of physical diagnosis was the core and pinnacle of our medical training. And it is an art. We benefited from being trained during the golden age of physical diagnosis. It remains the most important reason why South African physicians who emigrated, and who trained during this era, became so successful in which ever country they finally settled in. There were a few students who had natural talent, but most of us worked hard to acquire these skills.

Success at physical diagnosis requires a prodigious knowledge base, exquisite observational skills, the ability to sift though the chaff, and a sixth sense. Intuition. It is why all attempts to program computers for this task have failed so far. Computers might have a massive database, they can certainly sift through the trivial, but the subtle observational skills remain an issue. Perhaps the newest iterations of artificial intelligence will solve this, but I somehow doubt it — Star Trek notwithstanding. And if they develop intuition we could all be in trouble.

There were many role models to emulate and each had honed a different technique or approach.

These teachers are legendary in the annals of medical education at the University of Witwatersrand: Leo Schamroth, Asher Dubb, Mosie Suzman, Tom Bothwell, Harry Seftel. There was also a group of superb younger physicians, such as Mike Kew, who offered private evening and weekend tutorials. These were attended by all who had aspirations of becoming good doctors.

I first realized just what a different league these physicians played in, when I was on a ward-round with Mosie Suzman. Mosie was the husband of Helen Suzman, a prominent political figure who eventually became the only member of the Progressive Party in the South African Parliament. She was also the only real opposition against the ruling party. (And their niece, Janet Suzman became an award-winning film star in such movies as *Nicholas and Alexandra*.)

We had stopped by a bed in the large open ward, the standard lodging for the sick, and Mosie began examining a patient. He then turned to us and said, "In March 1958, over there in bed twelve was Mrs. Smith. She had a lovely smile. She presented with similar symptoms, but had disease X. And I recall a younger patient Miss Erasmus, who came to us from Potchefstroom after being misdiagnosed. She was in bed eighteen and we finally diagnosed her as having disease Y." It was evident that not only did he remember every patient he had ever seen, but he remembered every small detail of each patient. I was both in awe and totally intimidated by this level of recall. Some of us suspected there might have been a touch of performance art in his expositions, although none had the temerity to search through the hospital records to question his veracity. We took him at face value and learned from his wisdom.

More hours were spent in refining and perfecting our skills on how to take a good history and how to examine a patient than anything else during these years. Merely listening to the heart consumed days. One of the cardiologists produced a 33 rpm vinyl record of every conceivable heart sound — every click and murmur that emanated from each valve at all stages of the cardiac cycle. I listened to it for hours, occasionally interspersing it with a cut or two of the Beatles. Rheumatic fever was still a common condition, and the chronic effects of rheumatic heart disease was the bread and butter of cardiac diagnosis. So much so, that the inflammation it sometimes produced on the surface of the heart was known as "bread and butter pericarditis" — a sticky yellowish exudate. Rheumatic heart disease has all but disappeared, and imaging techniques such as echocardiography and angiography have completely replaced the stethoscope and the ear in figuring out heart anatomy. This is a very good thing, because I could never discern the various sounds especially when the heart was beating fast. No medical student today would waste precious time on such seeming trivia. They may not even listen to the Beatles.

One of the largest intellectual challenges was in the field of neurology. The first issue was evaluating the symptoms. The next was identifying the location of the defect or lesion in the brain or spinal cord. It was a diagnostic hybrid between geography (anatomy) and pathology.

A perfect example of this, was a unique disorder that had its roots on the crowded trains between the surrounding townships, like Soweto, and downtown Johannesburg. Gangsters on the train, sometimes known as "tsotsis" or "skellems" would use a sharpened bicycle spoke to stab commuters in the back as they stood crammed together. If done perfectly it damaged the spinal cord. Since the spoke was thin only half the cord would be transected. This resulted in paralysis on one side of the body and loss of temperature and pain sensation on the opposite side — also known as the Brown-Séquard syndrome, memorializing the physiologist who described it in 1850.

One morning we were instructed to examine a young woman with paralyzed legs — unable to stand or walk. During the examination, we noted that she had also lost all sensation on one side of her body. She could not detect light touch. Plunging needles into her skin elicited no response. Try as we could, we were unable to come up with a satisfactory diagnosis. It made no sense from any aspect of neuroanatomy. When the neurologist returned to hear our brilliant assessment, we moved down the ward to discuss the case. As we went over our evaluation and the demands it made on our knowledge, he quietly said, "Gentlemen, turn around now and tell me your diagnosis."

Our patient, who only moments before was lying paralyzed in bed, had put on a robe and was gaily walking to the bathroom at the end of the ward. We were dumbstruck. "Gentlemen," he said, "what you have just witnessed is a classic case of hysteria. The first clue is that the sensory loss was along a straight line. Nothing in nature is so perfectly straight. And the second clue is that the symptoms make no anatomical sense."

Words like hysteria are no longer acceptable, so today the diagnosis would be classified as a conversion disorder, a dissociative disorder, a somatoform disorder or the least objectionable phrase being a "functional neurological symptom disorder." These even have ICD codes so that insurance companies will authorize payment.

Such is the power of thought.

Chapter 21. Hot and Cold

Monday afternoon in the emergency department of "Non-European" Hospital, Hillbrow, adjacent to the medical school and catty corner to the whites-only Johannesburg General Hospital. "This patient has the concrete-pipe-syndrome", said the doctor. The patient had arrived in the emergency room in coma, blue and ice cold. The ER physician was using one of the many categorizations applied to a specific disorder, none of which would have been found in a standard medical book index. These were unique to South Africa, and often unique for a certain environment. The concrete-pipe-syndrome was the result of a weekend drinking bender, usually an African male between 20 and 70 years of age who was unable to find his way home after days of drinking, and who fell asleep in the nearest shelter, often an open concrete drainage pipe. The nights of Johannesburg winter could be chilly, sometimes falling below freezing. The combination of alcohol and cold exposure is potentially lethal.

This was not the only problem related to cold weather. Carbon monoxide poisoning was not uncommon, as coal stoves and oil space heaters supplied heat to some homes. Equally tragic were the burns, usually sustained by children, who grabbed hold of the red-hot heating bars of electric space heaters.

Of even greater significance was heat. The issue was not the lack of air conditioning, although that was a problem in homes and buildings, but the heat from the center of the Earth. South Africa has some of the deepest mines in the world, designed to extract minute amounts of gold from many tons of rock. Two miles underground the rock face reaches 140 degrees Fahrenheit. Working in such an environment is a challenge and engineers developed elaborate air conditioning and cooling systems to reduce the risk. Even so, not everyone's physiology is able to handle this.

One of our physiology field trips was to the Chamber of Mines laboratories associated with a large mining company. It was to impress upon us how the human body maintains a precise body temperature, and what occurs if it fails. Deep gold mining has many inherent dangers, but hyperthermia is at the top of the list. Working in the dark a mile underground, the temperature is in the nineties and large amounts of water are required to keep the dust down while drilling. The humidity is 100 percent. Being unable to cool off, despite dripping with sweat, it is easy to become both dehydrated and overheated.

The mines developed acclimatization chambers in which recent recruits could slowly adapt to the conditions they were about to face. These were the chambers awaiting our arrival. We stripped down to bathing trunks and sandals and entered the saunas. We were required to chart our vital signs, body weight and rectal temperature every ten minutes. We also had to collect our urine and measure its specific gravity. Actually this was hardly needed as a mere glance at it when the color resembled SAE 30 motor oil informed us that we were becoming dehydrated. Fortunately, the floors were covered with slatted and raised wooden floorboards, but within an hour the sweat almost submerged them, otherwise we might have needed scuba gear.

We were finally released once we had shed many pounds of water, our blood pressures had dropped, our pulses became thready and our body temperatures rose precipitously. None of us would have qualified for underground work.

I don't know what I learned from this experiment other than never wanting to live in Houston, Texas.

Chapter 22. Divination

It is hard to convey a sense of Dr. Harry Seftel with any fidelity. A tall string-bean of a man, whom his patients dubbed "the man who stands as high as the drip stand," he had an intensity and a contagious energy. When he spoke, he snapped out pithy phrases and observations like a machine gun, often accompanied by a spray of saliva for emphasis. They were brilliant salvos.

One day, while still students on his unit, a colleague presented a case of pneumonia during ward-rounds. I thought he did a credible job. Seftel then asked, "What did the sputum look and smell like?" The student meekly replied that he had not checked. Seftel picked up the metal sputum mug from the bedside stand, put it directly under the student's nose, snapped it open and snapped out. "My friend, medicine consists of secretions, concretions and excretions. Now smell!" I thought the student was going to pass out from the stench of the blue-green slime, the result of an organism known as Klebsiella.

"You don't need a laboratory to make a diagnosis, you need a nose." Seftel's reliance on the characteristics of sputum was legendary. On another occasion he picked up a sputum mug, raising it aloft like a trophy. "The mug is a crystal ball," he announced. We watched, stepped back a little and hoped he wouldn't spill anything. "Look inside, and you can predict the future." He lifted the lid and peered at the contents. "And the prediction is.........pulmonary TB!"

He insisted that we personally perform the examination on all body fluids — both chemical and microscopic. To him it was an integral part of the physical examination. No different from the patient's weight or temperature. There was a small laboratory bench and sink adjacent to the wards with all the glassware, stains and a microscope. His logic was flawless — "You care about your patient a lot more than some technologist in the laboratory down the hill. You want to make a diagnosis. They just want to finish their work." He was proved correct time and again when one of us would find a tuberculosis bacillus while the laboratory result was negative. Today, all that has changed. A nurses aide does the weighing, a nurse takes the temperature and a laboratory somewhere, sometimes in another state, examines the sputum. This is called modern healthcare — twice the cost for half the results.

He had elements of Sherlock Holmes, an exquisite skill of careful observation and brilliant synthesis. One day a 22-year-old, rural Xhosa female, was admitted to our unit, with a large, red, swollen knee. On ward-rounds in the morning I presented her case. He glanced at her, turned to me and said, "Benjamin, you do know the diagnosis, don't you?" "No sir," I said. "I was planning to get X-rays and some blood tests and examine the fluid in the knee joint today, sir." He looked down at me and remarked, "But you never commented on her toe-nails. Had you used your eyes and your brain, Benjamin, you would not need to waste any more time or money. This young lady has scurvy," he said, "and she has bled into her knee joint." "Her toenails are painted," he pointed out. "The only rural women who paint their nails are women of ill repute. And where do such women work? Obviously in bars (known as "shebeens" in Johannesburg). And where do they get their beer from? They brew it themselves in large iron pots. So the beer has lots of iron, and the iron gets absorbed and interferes with Vitamin C metabolism. And had you made her smile you would have noticed that her gums were bleeding. Now let's see if you can do any better with your next patient."

This ability of Dr. Seftel to understand and appreciate the cultural background of his patients was perhaps his biggest strength. Another patient, with one large bulging eye, was referred to us from a mission hospital. After a careful examination, I constructed a long list of possible diagnoses. The extent of one's differential diagnoses was often lauded, implying that one knew of all the many possibilities. On ward-rounds the next day, I proudly displayed my erudition and the various ways to get to the correct diagnosis. Seftel asked the patient a couple of questions, then looked at me and said, "Book the operating room tomorrow morning for a simple D and C — dilatation and curettage of the uterus." Seftel picked up my querulous expression.

Here was a patient with an eye problem and he was fussing with her uterus. "Benjamin," he said, "did you ask this young lady how many children she has." "Yes sir, she told me she had two." "And how many times has she been pregnant?" "I didn't ask that, sir." "Well had you asked, she would have said ten times. That means she has had at least eight miscarriages. And what is the most common cause of miscarriage in this rural population? TB of course. She has uterine TB and her eye is bulging because of a tuberculous tumor [tuberculoma] in the eye socket. The least invasive way to make the diagnosis is from her uterine lining."

Just another simple lesson from the maestro.

What follows is a brief selection of other "Seftelisms" as best as they can be re-called;

"I tell people not to smoke grass, but to eat grass."
The 5 S's of   Sickness — stuffing, stressing, sexing, smoking and sloth
Loudly announced to the entire ward after diagnosing gonorrhea in a patient.   *"Now we have to find all his contacts. This is when pubic health becomes public health."*
During a talk on nutrition:
"The breasts are no longer organs of nutrition. They have become organs of commerce and titillation."
"The only value in taking vitamins is to produce expensive urine."

"We are masters at death control, but not good at birth control."

"Any woman who smokes during pregnancy should be convicted of child abuse."

As mentioned, the local beer served in the illegal speakeasies ("shebeens") was home-brewed in iron pots. This resulted in large amounts of iron in the beer and for those who indulged in many gallons of beer each week an enormous intake of iron that was absorbed and deposited in various organs causing a variety of ills. Seftel referred to these patients as *"iron men in a gold city."*

Chapter 23. A Surgical Deity

By law and long-standing tradition, interns, or house-officers as they were known in South Africa, had to live within a quarter mile of the hospital so that they could respond to any emergency and be available when needed. This turned out to be all the time. Most of us lived in a building adjacent to the hospital, affectionately known as ResDoc. The accommodation was a small simple room with a bed, a table and a sink. The bathrooms were at the end of long corridors. On the first floor was the dining area. Across the road was the residence for the nursing school students, a fact that did not go unnoticed by the male interns. On the top floor of ResDoc were four small apartments for married couples. Such couples comprised only a tiny fraction of interns and were usually people who had begun medical school later in life, often after successful careers in other fields.

On day one of the surgical internship, we were summoned to be in Professor duPlessis' office at 6:30 am. This was the time he devoted to his house-officers. His registrars, roughly equivalent to residents in the USA, got the 7.00 am time slot, then came his junior consultants followed by the senior consultants.

In this era of surgical tyrants, it was no surprise that someone put a sign on his door announcing — "Tomorrow will be Thursday — God and Professor duPlessis willing." To his friends, whom we assumed he had some, he was known as "Sonny". To us he was simply "Doop".

Six newly minted interns, white coats freshly laundered, sat upright on the edge of our chairs. He looked us over and said, "Don't think that you are so smart or special. I can walk down Hospital Street and replace you with six interns as bright as you. And let me warn you, if you are ever in an argument with one of my nurses, you are wrong. I have spent twenty years training my staff. You are here for six months and then you are gone. Listen and learn from them." This set the tone for a memorable six months.

As a breed, surgeons have some striking characteristics — opinionated, brash, aggressive and forceful. He had all these features and then some. DuPlessis was a surgeon stereotype on steroids. On the other hand, his patients received the best care I ever witnessed throughout my medical life. Had I needed surgery I would have gladly selected his unit. With his patients he was surprisingly gentle and caring. To his staff he was a taskmaster. To his trainees, such as his house-officers, he was a martinet. It was also an undisguised secret that he believed there was no place for women in medicine — baby making and family distracting them from their duties. On the other hand he insisted on selecting the top six students in the graduating class for his interns. When a number of them were women one year, he put aside his misogyny, and all who wished were selected for his surgical unit. Intellectual elitism triumphed over prejudice.

He subscribed to the traditional methods of training and patient care, many going back to the precepts of predecessors like William Osler and Halsted. Our work schedule was supposed to be 36 hours on service or call and 12 hours off, perhaps one of the worst perversions inflicted on any form of training. Or patient care. Except he believed that if you had a really sick patient, you would remain available regardless of your schedule. We were not permitted to transfer the care of a complex or volatile situation to a colleague. This meant that we pretty much lived on the ward for the six months, catching occasional cat naps.

He also subscribed to the theory that one should be married to the profession, with no distractions. Getting married before one had completed all one's training was an anathema. Most surgeons were in the their thirties or early forties before contemplating marriage. I was the outlier. I also had no pretensions of becoming a surgeon. I had met my future spouse on Durban beach when I was seventeen, and we decided to get married during my internship. Our engagement was announced in the newspaper as was custom in those days. During the next "grand rounds", as duPlessis and his large entourage went from bed to bed, he finally resolved to congratulate me.

He put his hand on my shoulder, pronouncing loudly so all could hear, "Benjamin, you almost had a good career ahead of you."

Chapter 24. Glasses and a Pig

A firm believer in heroic surgery, Professor du Plessis — referred to as "Doop" — was fully committed to removing as much tissue as possible when operating on any form of cancer. The mantra at that time was to have the largest margin of normal tissue, without actually killing the patient. "You can't do microscopic removal for a microscopic disease" was the approach. All this has fortunately changed over the decades, and we are now able to do microscopic surgery. Of all the destructive and mutilating procedures, none was more so than the radical mastectomy for breast cancer.

One morning I was assisting "Doop" with a radical mastectomy. The patient was moderately obese with prodigious breasts. It was a warm day and there was no air conditioning in the hospital. He asked me to retract the breast tissue as he dissected it off the chest wall. I had to lean across the table to handle many pounds of jiggling breast tissue. I began to sweat, both from the heat and the protracted exertion. At the time I was wearing heavy tortoise shell glasses, and I felt them begin to slip down my nose. At the last second I flicked my head, but not in time. My glasses came off, brushed his arm and came to rest in the middle of the operative site. I jumped back, for fear that he was going to hit me. He took a large sterile swab, picked up my glasses and flung them into the corner of the room.

"We had better go and re-scrub and re-gown," he growled. I followed him into the scrub room and went to a sink as far from him as I could. His scrubbing ritual was interminable. I had learned to get a thick layer of foam and scrub just above the skin in the foam, otherwise my arms and hands would bleed. Nobody thought he believed that it was actually possible to physically remove every bacterium from the skin, but rather he was making a point about sterility. When we finally had our new gown and gloves we headed back into the operating room. "I am terribly sorry, sir," I said. "I only hope that you can see what the hell you are doing now," he grunted, my bloody glasses still lying on the floor. The anesthesiologist, who happened to be the head of the department, was almost purple from apoplectic laughter.

At the end of the case, I retrieved my glasses, washed them off and went to the nursing supply station. I got a roll of tape and taped the glasses to my entire face — nose, forehead, temples. When I went in for the next case, I looked like a baseball catcher. Within minutes, stories of this episode were being whispered around the hospital — such is the efficiency of the jungle telegraph.

This was not my only run-in with duPlessis in the operating room. I am about five foot eight inches on a good day. DuPlessis towered over me, being well over six feet. In the operating room he raised the table to the height he was comfortable with, a level in line with my chin. During one procedure, when I was on the same side of the table, he was continually getting his elbow in my face. Frustrated, he turned to the scrub nurse and said, "Goddam woman, get Benjamin a box to stand on." "He is already standing on one, sir," she responded. He turned to the registrar on the other side of the table and said, "It's time we stopped hiring these short-assed housemen."

The treatment for certain diseases, although seemingly logical at the time, now seems quite bizarre. Duodenal and gastric peptic ulcers were managed with bed rest, sedation and a constant supply of antacids, hopefully allowing the ulcers to heal. This was many years before two Australian pathologists recognized that a bacterium, *Helicobacter pylorii*, was the cause, for which they were awarded the Nobel Prize. The antacids were supplied through a nasogastric tube and milk was commonly used. It was put into a IV bottle and hung on an IV pole, being replaced every few hours as it slowly bathed the ulcer.

One day a patient was being wheeled out of the ward toward the operating room, when the head nurse noted that the IV bottle accompanying the patient was nearly empty. She called to a student nurse to put up a new bottle of IV fluid. The young nurse collected one from the refrigerator and hung a new bottle. The patient received about 100 ccs of whole, full cream milk intravenously before it was noticed. Remarkably, the patient did just fine, demonstrating the resilience of the human body — or the good quality of the milk.

Another novel therapy at the time involved pigs. Humans have many remarkable similarities to pigs — both species are omnivores, we share blood types, our skins are tightly attached to the underlying tissues, our antigens are similar so that we can partially tolerate transplants of pig skin and heart valves. Our behavior is comparable. The major difference is that they can't sweat which is why they roll around in liquids to cool off. It also turns out that pig liver works very much like ours. So for patients with acute liver damage, for example due to a virus or a toxin, a pig liver was used to tide them over for a while giving them a chance for their own liver to recover. The liver is a remarkably resilient organ and can regenerate cells rather quickly. This technique was designed some time before human-liver transplants became routine.

There was a menagerie on the roof of medical school, including a small baboon colony, housing for feral cats and stray dogs for the physiology and pharmacology departments, and then along came the pigs. When a pig liver was required, the job of pig catching was delegated to the intern. We were used to menial tasks. The major role of house-officers on ward-rounds was to pour tea for the consultants during the break. It was most certainly not to ever offer an opinion.

One evening I was informed that we were going to perform a "pig-liver-assist." DuPlessis still trusted my competence enough, despite dropping my glasses into the wound, to reward me with the task of catching a pig. As I chased the pig around its pen in the early hours of the morning, I couldn't help reflecting about my parents who had worked hard to support me going to medical school, and here I was, a pig catcher. Perhaps this would be the pinnacle of my career.

Chapter 25. Introduction to real death

Death is inevitable, a fact of life. Only in the USA do some families and physicians regard it as optional. Our introduction to a dead person was in the anatomy dissection halls. However, this was a sterile experience. We had not known the corpse during life, and the body had been pickled. There was no real connection, no emotional context. It was rather a metaphysical experience. And in short order, the remains that we confronted each day became just that — remains. It was muscles and fascia, vessels and nerves and organs. Thousands of names and places to memorize like a massive atlas.

The autopsies we witnessed during our year of pathology were similar. The patient was anonymous, and the brief case history presented prior to the examination of the organs was an aseptic accounting of desolate medical facts. The experience in the emergency room was much more intense, but the drama of events unfolded rapidly, and all the focus was on management. Some patients were dead on arrival or so near death that our ministrations were little more the medical last rites. It was easy to remain distant and detached from the person.

One of the rules in South Africa, perhaps even a law, was that only a physician could certify death, as if this required special training. This first came to my attention while a student at Baragwanath Hospital. I was on call for one of the general medicine wards, when my phone rang at two o'clock in the morning. "Doctor, Joe Shabalala is late." "I beg your pardon," I said. "Yes, doctor, Mr Shabalala is late." I am certainly not my sharpest during these witching hours, so I asked, "Late for what?" There was a little hesitation at the other end, and the nurse said, "No, doctor. Mr. Shabalala does not breathe any more." Then the penny dropped. The nurse was using a common euphemism that she had heard Europeans use when referring to a dear departed: "the late Mr. Smith."

During my surgical internship I cared for a delightful elderly lady with an obvious diagnosis of gastric obstruction. She could not tolerate any food. Although we suspected the worst, she underwent a laparotomy, but the stomach cancer had spread everywhere in her abdomen. There was a small side ward in which terminal patients could be kept in comfort and with some privacy. This was the leading edge of what eventually morphed into the hospice movement. This lady had no family, so every chance I had, I would drop by her room for a chat and to see her smile. After a number of days it was evident that she did not have much time left.

One day she said, "Dr. Benjamin, I am going to die tonight, but there is something I would like you to do for me. I would love a taste of my favorite food and drink — raw oysters and black velvet. Now I know that oysters are hard to come by, but I am sure you can find some champagne and Guinness stout." This combination, known as black velvet had been concocted in London to mourn the death of Prince Albert. It pairs beautifully with briny oysters.

That evening the two of us sat in her room drinking black velvets while she reminisced, occasionally falling in and out of sleep. Around three in the morning, she closed her eyes and stopped breathing. I sat there for a while before leaving the room to let the nurse know that she had died. As I reached for the door I heard a gasp. This agonal breathing went on for a couple of hours, the duration between gasps slowly getting longer.

Finally she was gone, as was the champagne.

Chapter 26. Expectations and traditions.

Surgery grand rounds were held every Saturday morning. Professor duPlessis, the head of the surgery department, led the parade from patient to patient, pontificating over some key observation after the house officer succinctly presented the case to the group. Strict protocol was followed. It was similar to our initial introduction to surgery. Closest to the boss was the head nurse, clutching a clipboard and pad for notes and instructions. The senior consultants clustered around, all hoping that one day they, too, would have a surgical unit of their own. Then came the junior consultants whose future was questionable, unless there was a mass die-off of those above them. Registrars followed, with house officers and medical students at the periphery, hoping to catch a few nuggets of surgical wisdom, while on tenterhooks that they would be selected for interrogation.

This was followed by the inevitable morning tea and a presentation of the discharge summaries for patients sent home the previous week. Each house officer prepared a concise and condensed summary of every key fact about the patient, usually on a single page. The chart was culled of all extraneous paper and other information not deemed worthy of saving. Everything was bound into a small booklet of sorts. Should the patient be readmitted for any reason, a mere glance at the discharge summary would contain all the pertinent information. No paging through screeds of useless documents. These discharge summaries were perfectly designed for patient care, not for malpractice attorneys. In fact, the latter concern never entered into the equation, nor were there volumes of legal requirements. DuPlessis read every word in each discharge summary and only when he was completely satisfied were we dismissed for the rest of the day. Some Saturdays we did not leave until after sunset.

There were two long-standing traditions during the last week of the surgery internship. The house-officers were expected to take the professor and his entire surgical retinue out for a farewell dinner. Since I was already becoming a foodie I selected the restaurant — a good French place with an awful name, the Linger Longer. We seated duPlessis at the head of the table. I was to his right. For my first course I ordered snails. I caught a glimpse of curiosity on his face as if to ask, "What does a surgical house-officer know about this kind of food?" The dish was delivered — a classic preparation, the garlic wafting ahead of its arrival. I picked up the first shell with the tongs, perhaps hoping to impress him with my expertise, but failed to grasp the entire thing. The tongs snapped shut, launching my snail across the table. It hit duPlessis in his midriff, garlic-butter-parsley dripping down his expensive silk tie. This was the last time I had to apologize to him.

The second tradition was played out on the last day of the internship. It was receiving "grades" for our performance over the six months. They were presented in the form of a book. The book that duPlessis chose that year was *The Student Life* written by Sir William Osler. It was the philosophy we were instructed to follow.

This is how the grades worked - no book, an F; a book, an E: a signed book, a C; a wrapped signed book, a B: and finally a wrapped signed book with some brief comment on the fly page, an A.

I still treasure my copy.

Chapter 27. Children

Following the mandatory internship year of general surgery and medicine we were deemed responsible enough to care for women and children. Six months of pediatrics and another half year in obstetrics seemed the appropriate path to pursue, because at that stage I had no idea what I wanted to do when I grew up. I had forsaken a career in the basic sciences, and some aspects of clinical medicine were still enticing.

I was beginning to discern a significant flaw in my personality. While I cared deeply about my patients and was determined to provide the best possible care, I lacked empathy for people who had abused themselves, intentionally or not. This was not a pleasant revelation. I had entered medicine with the firm intention of helping humanity, regardless of any individual's circumstance — the typical naiveté of youth. I got irritated when awakened at three o'clock in the morning to look after an obese alcoholic who smoked two packs of cigarettes a day and was wandering around the ward with delirium tremens peeing on his neighbors and cursing the nurses. A vague uneasiness began creeping over me about the constant demands that others were making on my life and my lack of any control. I put that all aside when I went 'down the hill' to the Transvaal Memorial Hospital for Children. I imagined that I would have none of those feelings working with innocent children, ignoring the reality that most children come with parents.

Solly Levine, the chief pediatrician, was the Seftel of pediatrics. Where Seftel used the sputum mug to divine diagnoses, Levine used the contents of the diapers. The British medical journal *Lancet* published one of his articles titled "The art of stool gazing", decrying the fact that most physicians no longer examined this evidence closely. Back in those days, pediatrics was a real specialty, as most infants and children were well cared for by the local family doctor, a general practitioner. Only in the most serious cases which the GP could not manage was the pediatrician consulted. And those youngsters who landed up in a children's hospital were especially heartbreaking.

Most childhood cancers were both untreatable and rapidly fatal. Rheumatic fever was epidemic, destroying hearts and lives. Congenitally acquired infections, such as those due to cytomegalovirus or German measles did irrevocable damage to the brain and other organs. Fortunately, by then the polio vaccine had eliminated the paralysis scourge that we had lived with when we were children, but complications from other infections were commonplace. Most congenital heart anomalies could not be surgically repaired.

Day after day we dealt with existential questions and difficult decisions. None was worse than the management of premature babies. Because of very limited resources, there were only two infant ventilators in the premie unit. There was a daily prioritization about which infant might benefit the most. A set of criteria was established, guidelines for who might live and who would probably die. There were times we had to remove an infant from a ventilator, because in our judgement another infant might have a greater chance of survival. This was not regarded as playing God, it was dealing with reality.

We had been taught that approximately 70% of any diagnosis was the result of taking a good history, about 20% was by performing a thorough physical examination; the small remainder was gleaned from the results of ancillary tests — x-rays, laboratory tests on various body fluids and such. Pediatrics resembles veterinary medicine, as many patients cannot provide a history. Reliance is placed on the parents or other care givers to tell the story. The quality of this history was dependent on the observational skills of the parent overlain by many other factors — educational background, economics, cultural and social factors, family dynamics and many others. The skill of the pediatrician was in deciphering the information — what was valid, what was exaggerated, what was being hidden or withheld. One learned to never discount a parent's observation. One did so at one's peril. That being so, conducting a sensitive and compassionate interrogation was a high art, a skill granted only to the favored few. I ranked myself in the average category.

I watched families torn asunder and marriages disintegrate as parents struggled to deal with the exigencies of their offspring's health problems. It was emotionally draining, compounded by the call schedule of 36 hours on and 12 off. One functioned in a perpetual foggy daze. Most disconcerting was waking in the morning, knowing that you had responded to a half dozen calls during the night and not remembering what treatments you had sanctioned or recommended.

The hope was that you avoided some serious blunder.

28. Culture, Sociology and Medicine

The importance of understanding the social and cultural characteristics of one's patients was constantly reinforced. Perhaps the most dramatic example was a lesson we learned from a shaman — a traditional healer. Much to the chagrin of his Zulu tribe, Vasamazulu C Mutwa had written a major treatise on their mythology and history — *Indaba, my children*. It caused quite a stir when published. To this day I only retain three books from South Africa - *Jock of the Bushveld, Cry, the Beloved Country* and *Indaba, my children*.

Mutwa was invited to accompany us on ward rounds at Baragwanath Hospital near the black township of Soweto. After examining a half dozen patients we stopped for the traditional morning tea break and chatted about various issues. One of the patients we had seen with heart failure had recently been re-admitted with digitalis toxicity. This was the drug most commonly used in managing a less than energetic heart. Toxicity to this medication was common in this population. Mutwa asked to see an example of a digitalis pill. We handed him a bottle with dozens of tiny pills. He shook his head and then with a sad smile, said, "You have just told a patient that his heart, the most important and vital part of his body is sick, and then you tell him to take one tiny pill a day. What do think he is going to do? Why don't you get the pharmacy to reformulate it in a large tablet, big enough for a horse. That will solve this problem." He then repeated one of the aphorisms of Zulu medicine, which has been known to many cultures for millennia: *"you can't treat an evil disease with a sweet medicine."*

Hospitals in South Africa reflected the same extreme racial separation as everything else in the society. There were places where wealthy whites, or those with insurance, could go to avoid the long waits and indignities of the hospitals like the Johannesburg General Hospital, funded by the provincial government. Catering to this elite were institutions that used the word "clinic" to differentiate themselves from the masses. The major hospital serving the black population was Baragwanath, on the edge of Soweto (South Western Township), an area of over a 1 million people, linked to the heart of Johannesburg by trains, green buses operated by the Public Utility Transport Corporation (PUTCO) and numerous unregistered and usually unlicensed taxis.

Baragwanath Hospital — or simply "Bara" as it was commonly called, is the third largest hospital in the world, with over 3000 beds sprawling across 172 acres. The name is not indigenous, but was named after a Cornish immigrant whose Welsh name was derived from bara (wheat) and gwanath (bread) and who had built a small inn near the current site of this behemoth. It was originally constructed as a military hospital and paid for by the United Kingdom, primarily to serve troops and for the convalescence of wounded soldiers from the Second World War. This is reflected in its barracks-style design, with large general wards linked with walkways and separated by open spaces. It was so large that one had to drive from the medical student/physician housing area to the operating room or the emergency department. As a bonus, it had some recreational facilities for the staff.

Adjacent to medical school in central Johannesburg was the Non-European hospital (NEH) devoted to a different demographic. This is where those considered not worthy of treatment at the "Gen" were consigned, including Indians (both Hindu and Muslim), Chinese, Coloreds and a small select group of patients referred to the big city from mission or other rural hospitals for specialty care. It also managed acute emergencies for inner city Bantu who might not have survived transport to Bara. During this time the government, in its infinite wisdom and deep knowledge of racial differences, declared that Japanese were white. This was a convenient political move, as there were no Japanese in the country, but South Africa had begun to trade with Japan and wished to develop a diplomatic relationship. NEH had a superb nursing and medical staff and was a premier facility for the training of medical students.

Another provincially operated teaching facility on the edge of town was Coronation Hospital. This served the Indian and Colored population. For those who did not grow up in the bizarre racial milieu of South Africa, the word "Colored" may sound pejorative, but it is not. It is a term applied to a very distinctive multi-ethnic subgroup who were the most cosmopolitan of racial hybrids — a mix of Dutch whites, Khoisan (Bushmen and Hottentots), Bantu, Malay and other South Asians. As one might suspect, this was a result of some miscegenation and DNA mixing in the early days of South Africa, largely in the

Cape province. *Homo sapiens* is a particularly promiscuous species. Such mixed-race people did not fit neatly into the major groups and were largely shunned by both Europeans and Bantu, resulting in a unique and distinctive culture. They are mainly Afrikaans speakers, although with many of their own expressions and idioms, and they show an amazing blend of physical characteristics.

Our training included stints at all these hospitals. Each had a singular mix of patients and pathologies, but all had wonderful clinical staff. One evening a colleague and I drove to Coronation Hospital to begin a surgical rotation. For reasons that were never elucidated, young Colored women bent on committing suicide did it by drinking lye. Perhaps it was no more than its ready availability. Unfortunately, lye causes severe burns in the mouth, and especially the esophagus. Many survived the initial insult, but over the ensuing months the esophagus became progressively scarred and useless. Without some form of surgical repair the final outcome was starvation. To deal with this the surgeons at Coronation had devised a procedure to replace the burnt and scarred areas of the gullet with a segment of the patient's large intestine. This was not a trivial procedure, and we were on our way to assist at one of these major surgical interventions.

Even during this period in the 1960s Johannesburg had a high crime rate. Houses had burglar proofing over the windows, and doors were always locked. In Durban and Capetown, on the other hand, crime was quite uncommon. Even so, Johannesburg was a far cry from what it eventually became — one of the most dangerous cities in the world. In addition to the crime, driving was another serious hazard. This was a result of many old, poorly maintained vehicles, unlicensed drivers and the usual combination of alcohol, drugs and lack of sleep. Because of this, and the habit of many drivers who attempted to beat a changing traffic light, I always hesitated for a few second after the light turned green before accelerating into the intersection.

On the way to Coronation we stopped at an traffic circle near the Lever Brothers factory. I waited a few seconds after the light changed. It was not enough time. A 1948 Desoto came barreling through the red light at about 60 miles a hour. Fortunately, I glanced it coming on my periphery and braked hard. In an instant, the entire front end of the turquoise

Ford Prefect that my mother had donated to me disappeared. It was carried on the front of the Desoto, smashing into the entrance gate of the factory. The doors sprung open, and a dozen individuals fled into the darkness. When the driver, noticeably shaken, was asked by the police for his license, he produced a scrap of paper that was an old, expired learner's license. His "taxi" was also illegal. Despite the carnage, no one was seriously injured. We did not make it to the hospital that evening so I never learned the details of that esophageal replacement operation. Since surgery was not in my future and being unlikely to encounter this particular issue again, it saved space in my memory circuits for other topics.

Medical students, especially in their senior years, were given a great deal of responsibility for the management of patients, from the simple suturing of lacerations, to the insertion of chest tubes to drain blood or pus, or to allow the lung to expand. At Bara we were taught how to do circumcisions on adolescents or young adults. The practice of ritual circumcision in the black population at or even after puberty was commonplace and was usually conducted in less than sanitary conditions, with instruments that were partially blunt or rusty and

146

without any anesthetic. As you might imagine, the young men did not look forward to this procedure, so we offered a suitable alternative. We gave a local anesthetic in a ring pattern around the base of the penis, ensuring that the important nerves were blocked, and then proceeded with the trimming.

Some Africans are genetically predisposed to develop considerable scarring around superficial injuries, forming ugly nodules of fibrous tissue known as keloids, and we always hoped this would not occur. Keloids could follow something as innocuous as ear piercing, or any surgical procedure. Evidently, one young man developed a great deal of keloid scar tissue in the months following his circumcision. To our dismay he was not disappointed or upset with the results. He even recommended the same procedure to his friends. In the USA it would have probably resulted in a lawsuit, not accolades for the medical profession.

If there was any benefit in the apartheid system for our education, it underlined the uniqueness of each ethnic group and each individual. We had to understand how they viewed health and disease, and what therapeutic approaches to pursue, carefully tailoring history taking and the physical examination. This included knowledge of the tribe, language, religion, sex, education level, socio-economic status, work history and many other factors. During my general medicine internship, this was reinforced daily.

Our training never fell victim to the erroneous idea that there was a dichotomy between the mind and body. The best treatment was the one that helped the patient, even if we didn't understand scientifically how it worked. Using a placebo was entirely acceptable. With the advances in neurobiology, we are finally beginning to get an inkling of these relationships, although there is still a great deal to be learned.

We always questioned patients about the treatments they had received prior to coming to us. A sizable majority paid visits to their local healer, and only when they failed to improve or worsened did they consider western medicine. Since the majority of maladies are self limited or improve without any intervention, regardless of the incantations or medications administered by the *inyanga* (herbalist), by the time a patient came to us, they were often seriously ill. Unfortunately certain "medications" used by the *inyangas* were potentially toxic, especially the salts of heavy metals like cadmium. We kept a selection of these various powders and concoctions in a box and asked patients to point out what they had taken.

Non-European Hospital was where East Indians, both Hindu and Muslim, received hospital care. Family members were always at the bedside. The family also provided all the food for their hospitalized loved one. As house officers we got to know each family well. When it became known that I enjoyed Indian cuisine, I was kept well supplied with samosas, pakoras, various chaats and all manner of naan. We received invitations to family weddings and other celebrations. Fortunately, cell phones had not yet been invented, otherwise we would have spent entire days answering questions and communicating with members of a patient's family.

In today's hospitals in the USA, family members are encouraged to stay at the bedside around the clock, but for different reasons. They are there to protect their loved ones from a system that has become so fractured that errors in communication between staff have created a dangerous environment.

And the hospital food remains just as bad.

Chapter 29. Formality, dress codes and standards

Minutes after beginning an erudite sermon on some critical topic of general surgery, Professor duPlessis paused, making a soft off-screen comment to one of the female students in the front row. She abruptly rose and left the lecture. Turned out, she was not wearing stockings — perhaps because she was wearing sandals, an even more egregious misdemeanor.

The dress code was not a formal document, but widely understood and strictly observed. If in doubt, the head nurse or hospital matron was a reliable source of guidance. On the first day of their six month stint as house-officers (aka interns) with the Chief of Surgery, the two women in the elite group were informed that stockings and skirts was the standard kit beneath their laboratory coats. The nursing students on the ward were expected to wear black stockings and black lace-up shoes.

The men wore clean white laboratory coats and ties with muted colors and designs. Solids or simple stripes were favored. I recall Dr. Harry Seftel railing against visiting American medical students who arrived on his ward without neckties. He snapped, "We dress properly out of respect for our patients."

A major conflict erupted late in our training when we approached the provincial hospital administration and the medical school requesting permission to wear white pants and white safari jackets, especially in summer. The trend had begun in fancy private medical offices as a way to survive the heat, as air conditioning, like television, had not yet reached the country. Weeks of negotiation ensued before we were victorious, although some of the units still insisted on tradition.

The dress mirrored the deferential relationship that students had with medical school faculty. "Sir," was the expected appellation for men and "doctor" or "professor" was used when addressing the female faculty. As students, we were addressed as Mister or Miss, occasionally just by our surname if we were about to be humiliated. After graduation we finally earned the "doctor" title. Seldom did a student or house-officer initiate a conversation with staff or faculty. We were to be seen, not heard.

Behind this facade of formality there was intense caring and respect for one another. This may seem counterintuitive, but I was constantly surprised how much the faculty knew about each of us. I recall a meeting with the dean who made some of the most astounding comments and observations about my friends, my social life and extracurricular activities. I had befriended his beautiful young secretary of Greek heritage, and she mentioned that before he met with any student he would review their file so that he was fully prepared. This was reminiscent of Lord Mountbatten. When he received his first naval commission, he spent the night before meeting his crew reviewing every file of over one hundred men. After being piped aboard, he went down the line greeting each man by name and making some brief personal comment.

This begs the question how the information about each of us was obtained. I don't believe that the South African Secret Police, which was known to be very effective, worked for the University. There must have been some other underground source. Perhaps the original Deep Throats.

All this formality was brought into sharp contrast on arrival in Seattle at the University of Washington. Dress was casual, ties and jackets were eschewed and the town was rapidly descending into a fashion that eventually became known as grunge. Everyone was addressed by their first name creating a superficiality of friendship or at least camaraderie. In reality this was barely skin deep. It was sloppy. And it spilled over into performance.

In South Africa, just as we were expected to have standards of dress and social interaction, so were we expected to meet the very high standards of academic achievement and clinical performance. Anything less was frowned upon. Failure meant finding another occupation. On the other hand I never heard of an American medical student not graduating or becoming certified once they were accepted into a training program. Years later, after joining the faculty at a the University of Washington, I refused to certify the time that a resident spent with us at Children's' Hospital. His performance was poor and I felt strongly that he would not be a good diagnostician. To complicate matters he was the son of a faculty member. The chairman of the department called me to discuss the matter. "Denis," he said, "he is going into research. He doesn't want to do any clinical work." "In that case," I said, "he doesn't need any clinical certification."

There was a serious downside to the paradigm of care that people like Professor duPlessis both modeled and demanded. While the care provided to patients was exemplary, for the caregiver it was all-consuming — an all or nothing approach. Knowing instinctively that if one wasn't willing to devote every waking, and dreaming moment to one's patients, they were not receiving optimal care. That was unacceptable.

For the eclectic, aware that there were many other things in life outside of medicine, this model of care and caring was very difficult to live up to. The expectation was set so high, and I was unwilling to reach it. Du Plessis was correct when he suggested that I might have had a good career had I not got married. While I loved medicine and science in general, I had too many other interests to be this one-dimensional, totally devoted to a single "mistress."

Many of my colleagues readily adopted this model and ethic of caring. Combined with the superb training in clinical diagnosis, it was yet another important reason they were so successful in their professions and why this generation of physicians who went abroad developed a reputation of clinical excellence. I envied my friends who developed such single minded devotion.

Grading examinations was another area where we diverged from the American system. The body of knowledge required for a physician is immense. No one can know everything. Not even close. This was accepted as a fact. There was no illusion of perfection. Instead it was a stimulus to keep learning. For us a passing grade was a C, suggesting that one knew about half of what is known. A small number of individuals were awarded with a B, and the rare person was given an A. There was an appreciation that most people were average. The grading system followed the typical Gaussian distribution curve — the majority in the middle, and a few at either end.

In the USA, on the other hand, "grade creep" resulted in a curve skewed to the far right. Everyone expects to be exceptional. Any score less than 90% was met with protests. I was unaware of this perversion until I graded an examination for medical technology students during my first year on the faculty. I knew nothing of the concept of a 4.0 grade average. I still don't. Following this particular examination, there was mass outrage. Students were in tears outside my office door. Some had never received less than an A. I was told that their future, job prospects and careers would forever be tainted by a low grade. The head of the department called me into his office and gave me a tutorial about the grading system. It was a revelation and not a particularity good one. I was labeled as the meanest, stingiest tutor in the department. It did not take me long to fall in line and adapt to this new reality. I had no idea that I was training the most brilliant and knowledgeable students on the planet, but according to my grades they were almost perfect.

Another disparity related to scientific rigor and publication. In South Africa being published in the scientific literature was regarded as a sacred act. As such, it had to meet any number of stringent requirements. Firstly, it had to add something significant to the body of knowledge, not some trivial observation. The science, logic, statistics and research had to be beyond reproach. The manuscript went through multiple reviews at all levels in the hierarchy with final approval by the department chairperson. None of these reviewers expected to add their names to the author list. They were merely performing due diligence. There was no mandate to publish — no publish or perish ethic. Faculty were judged on their clinical skills and teaching abilities. Publishing was an important bonus, but not their raison d'être.

In the USA one would be hard-pressed to identify a junior person's mentor. Some department heads no longer critically review what their acolytes write or present, although they often append their name to the tail of a long author list. In most places it is a free-for-all, with little oversight, standards or significant editing. When I became an editor of a subspecialty journal, this level of sloppiness was all too obvious. Had I had my way, our journal would have only accepted a tiny fraction of the manuscripts that reached my desk, but that would have reduced the number of issues to one every couple of years. Unfortunately, we were expected to produce six issues a year with a minimum number of pages, so it became filled with the trivial or irrelevant, like so much of the so-called "medical literature." Worse than publishing meaningless studies, we followed up to find out what happened to all those articles we rejected because of questionable science. To no one's surprise, almost all were published in other journals.

Chapter 30. Serendipity

I stumbled exhausted into the doctor's dining room at the Children's Hospital room around 7 am to get a reviving cup of coffee, my face grizzly with a two-day beard. I had been on call for 36 hours and during the night had admitted 12 children, few of whom needed to be in hospital. As house-officers, we had no power to countermand the decision of the emergency room physician. I had also fielded all the calls that night, being the only on-call intern for the entire hospital. Between interviewing parents, doing physical examinations, writing notes, nurses would call worried that little Joey was turning blue or Mary's wheeze was getting worse.

After inhaling the insipid brew, I went to the bathroom to straighten up and prepare for early morning ward-rounds. Once I had given all my reports, I was free to leave and find a bed. But I knew it might be noon before all was straightened out after the previous evening's tsunami of patients. In the mirror was a barely recognizable face — bleary sunken eyes, sallow skin. "This is not fun," I thought. "This is not how I want to spend the rest of my life."

The next day I called Dr. Harry Seftel, my sensei, and asked for an appointment. "Benjamin," he asked, "what would you really like to do with your life?" "I would like to be involved in international health," I responded. "In that case, you need to get a Masters degree. Consider going to a place like the London School of Hygiene and Tropical Medicine." As intrigued as I was, I could not face another two to three years of training, especially under the British system, as effective as it is. I am a rebel at heart and needed some independence. Enough humiliation and put downs.

I puzzled about my future. I needed a profession where I had some control over my own life. Much to my surprise, the thought of pathology kept coming back. I had hated pathology as a medical student, and I had spent years working towards a career in clinical medicine. Making the psychological switch did not come easily. But I knew that I was a pretty good microscopist, and I had enjoyed the year of clinical pathology or what later became known as laboratory medicine.

I began exploring training programs in the USA. The Harvard affiliated hospitals in Boston and

Stanford stood out as highlights. Ex-pat South Africans had excelled at both. I began writing letters and making inquiries. I met with Professor duPlessis who recommended Washington University in St. Louis. The head of surgical pathology there, Dr. Laurin Ackerman, had recently spent a year-long sabbatical in South Africa. He was a legendary teacher, and author of the standard textbook on the subject. Back then, St. Louis did not have a wonderful reputation, and lifestyle was as important to me as was the training. To my shock, I received an acceptance letter from Washington University without ever having applied. Evidently, duPlessis had recommended me to Ackerman, proving the old adage that "it is not what you know, it is who you know." Writing a "thanks, but no thanks" letter was not easy.

The Southern states of the USA were also expunged off my list, for the same reasons that I was leaving South Africa. The East Coast schools all seemed too stuffy, too hide-bound by tradition, still clinging to the formality of the motherland. From reports, the Midwest sounded gruesome. A cousin of mine who had gone to Chicago was mugged during the first month. By exclusion, that left the west. I had never heard of Oregon, and Washington was a mystery. That left the allure of California. Even though California made it especially difficult for foreign medical graduates, a number of South Africans were successfully thriving there. With great anticipation, I sent an application to Stanford for the 1971 academic year. My plan was to do a senior house-job in obstetrics and spend at least six months traveling, before embarking on the next stage of my education and training. I waited for the response, and waited and waited.

Panicking, I consulted with Professor Tom Bothwell, Chairman of Medicine. He had an international reputation and one assumed that he had good insights and contacts. As I was sitting in his waiting room, a registrar I had once worked with, Dr. Peter Jacobs, came in. He had recently returned from a yearlong fellowship in the USA. We chatted about my plight and he said, "Go to Seattle, the University of Washington." "Never heard of it," I said. "It's a great little place, and the young university and medical school is exceptional." It also turned out that Bothwell and the head of hematology at the University of Washington had collaborated for many years on iron metabolism research.

That evening Vivien and I looked up Seattle in the *Encyclopedia Brittanica*. There was a short entry stating that Seattle was a center for the timber industry, fishing and aerospace. One small photograph of two golfers under an umbrella with Mt. Rainier in the distance was the only visual. It seemed like an interesting option, and I sent in an application. To my astonishment I received a phone call a few weeks later, not only offering me a position in the residency program, but asking if I could begin in the 1970 academic year. I decided to accept and negotiated a contract giving us only a couple of months to travel in Europe.

About a month later I received an acceptance letter from Stanford. The departmental secretary had put a 6-cent stamp on the envelope, and it had gone surface mail via mail ship taking almost three months to reach me.

This underscored an aphorism that became my mantra. "Life is planned serendipity, and the planning doesn't matter."

Chapter 31. A New Life

As soon as I signed the contract for a residency in pathology at the University of Washington in Seattle, we organized to leave South Africa, a full year before our initial plans. Getting rid of stuff was easy as we had very little stuff — a bed and two cars. I drove my small, third hand Fiat to a second hand car dealer — a term that has been replaced with the euphemism pre-owned, as if that will hide the fact that the vehicle had been abused and poorly maintained. The dealer glanced at the car and said, "How much will you pay me to take your car?" I drove it to the junk yard.

We packed up a few unopened wedding presents, mainly unneeded stainless steel things, some treasured books and an antique brass microscope that my grandfather had gifted to me. It all occupied a small crate that was shipped to Seattle to arrive some time after our arrival. South Africa had stringent restrictions on taking money out of the country — about 2000 Rand, which at the time translated to roughly a little over $2000. Since that was about all we had, I borrowed money from my grandfather for the airline tickets, promising to pay him back as soon as I earned a stipend.

We left without much fanfare spending two months in Europe, where we managed to travel on $5 a day. Needless to say we did not eat in Michelin star restaurants. In Italy we would walk across town to save 100 lire — a few cents — for a meal. In the week prior to our departure Vivien broke a knuckle during a field hockey game, leaving me to do most of the heavy lifting which was not much of a problem as we had little luggage and nothing heavy.

A conscious decision was made to fly directly from London to Seattle, avoiding the expected indignities of New York. We had obtained exchange visitors visas, as the Vietnam War was in full stride. Had we applied for permanent residency, I could have been drafted, inducted into the army, shipped to Vietnam, killed and finally arrived in the USA in a body bag.

On arrival in Seattle, the company responsible for transportation from the airport to the city was on strike. The only option was a taxi, which neither of us had ever used before. We had reservations at an inexpensive apartment hotel in the university district and handed the address to the cab driver. We mentioned to him our reason for being in Seattle. He asked, "Are you in a rush or do you have some time?" As there was no urgency to get anywhere, we said we had time. He turned off the meter and said, "In that case I will give you a tour of your new home." For the next hour he drove us all over the city, introducing us to the major areas and landmarks. It was instant love.

Then began the adaptation, the learning of new ways and very strange habits. We knew that we needed a car. With the money we had saved we paid cash for a Ford Maverick of a bronze color that went by the cute name of freudian gilt. We found a small "furnished" apartment near Green Lake, a few miles from the medical school and University Hospital. What we didn't' appreciate was what the word "furnished" meant. In South Africa, this implied furniture, a fully equipped kitchen, linens, towels, bedding. All we discovered was a bed, a table, a couple chairs, a refrigerator and a stove. Being frugal out of necessity, we went to the nearest Goodwill store and bought two of everything we needed. The two dinner plates cost a dime apiece, and fifty years later we still have them. By now they could be valuable antiques.

The waitress at the diner where we first breakfasted had to explain bizarre phrases like "over easy" and "sunny side up" while I insisted that I just wanted a couple of fried eggs. And our first visit to a supermarket was both a revelation and terrifying. In South Africa we had the choice of two breads — white or brown. These were stacked like cord wood and never wrapped or packaged; one picked up a loaf with a square of waxed paper or thin parchment paper. In Seattle we discovered an entire aisle of breads, many made with grains we had never heard of. Even more daunting were the breakfast cereals. The choice was overwhelming. We had no idea there were that many ways to foist large amounts of sugar on the public. When we reached the checkout our basket was almost empty and Vivien was in tears. " I have no idea what to choose," she said, "and even if I did we can't afford it."

Of all the adaptations, the issue of choice was the most striking. But the choice was for food products no person concerned about nutrition would want. Is there really a need for a hundred different cereals or thirty varieties of spaghetti sauce? On the other hand the choice of fruit, vegetables and meats was a mere fraction of what we were accustomed to. Where was the tongue, the kidneys, the sweetbreads, the lamb breasts? The contrast between manufactured food and real food was stark. Back then there were only three varieties apples, red delicious, golden delicious and Granny Smith. They looked beautiful, but suffered dearly from their time in cold storage. Things have improved a little over the years, although real food still occupies a tiny fraction of the periphery of the supermarket, while the rest comes from a factory.

After moving into our little "furnished" apartment, the next revelation was arranging for a telephone installation. In South Africa that might have taken a number of years and a few bribes. We received an apology that the technician would be delayed for a day. And what color phone did we want? Color? Color? In South Africa the choice was between black or black. I was at work the day the technician arrived to install and hook up the phone. Vivien was so desperate for conversation with someone other than me, that she spent a couple of hours speaking to the serviceman. Many months later we happened to bump into the technician at a party. He immediately recognized Vivien, and commented that he had never before been cornered for such a long conversation with a customer.

Today we no longer have a landline telephone.

Chapter 32. Seattle 1970

As was promised in the *Encyclopedia Britannica*, Seattle in 1970 was still a small provincial town, barely clinging to the edge of the continent. Boeing and the University of Washington were the major employers. Truck farms with fresh produce, and the best strawberries on earth, were fifteen minutes from downtown. Traffic was unheard of. I could drive to the Pike Street market from the hospital in ten minutes and find parking. There were so few visitors to the city and its downtown market that serious consideration was given to tearing the old structure down, and building office towers. The contrast to Johannesburg was especially striking.

When we left Johannesburg it was already a large, bustling cosmopolitan city. It was ethnically diverse with vibrant immigrant communities. The black population was consigned to the large township slums on the edge of the city, or in backyard "servants quarters," — single concrete rooms to which they could repair after a long day of service — cleaning, cooking, gardening, baby-sitting.

Johannesburg had many restaurants, reflecting its international population. Crime was already a problem, but we all learnt street smarts in early childhood. By the age of ten I was able to take the bus downtown on my own to get my braces tightened at the dentist, and felt comfortable enough to walk twenty blocks to my father's business for a ride home. As teenagers, hitch-hiking was an acceptable mode of transportation.

Seattle in the 1970s was not diverse — dominated by a cold, distant, population of blond Norwegians and Swedes. A small black population occupied a ghetto on the edge of downtown, near the artlessly named International District, the home of the Chinese with competing dim sum restaurants. For the most part, the white population was desperately middles class, but intermixed with the moneyed, who occupied the opulent homes on the view side of the street. These were the banking mavens, the forestry robber barons, and the aerospace executives.

Starbucks was already there — a tiny shop hidden in the market, catering to a small immigrant population who wanted whole beans and knew how to grind coffee. Everyone else was drinking Folgers

Crystals or Yuban. It remained that way for thirty years. Nordstrom was an inconspicuous family shoe store. REI sold a few climbing ropes, crampons, carabiners, and some camping equipment. The restaurants were poor, unless one was addicted to deep fried dishes. There were a few high class places, which we could not afford, and still can't.

Most remarkable, was that salmon still entered the waterways in large numbers during the late summer and fall runs. A resident colleague and I borrowed a rubber boat. After work one afternoon we launched it into the "cut" — a channel between Lake Washington and Lake Union. Within an hour we had our limit of sockeye salmon. (Today it is unlikely that my grandchildren will ever know the taste of wild salmon).

A medical school friend visited us a year after our arrival. I was insulted that he referred to Seattle as "this little hick town." In retrospect he was correct, but we fell in love with it. The worst part was that it did not stay that way. Our first fifteen years in the Pacific Northwest were magical, introducing us to the great outdoors — hiking, skiing, sailboat racing, clamming, crabbing, mushroom hunting, gardening, wild food foraging, fishing, and eventually hunting. I learned ikebana from a Japanese teacher and even toyed with bonsai.

Then it all changed. We began a family, and Seattle grew up.

Chapter 33. Sitting at the feet of giants

We knew little about Seattle, apart from the entry in the *Encyclopedia Britannica*, even less about the University of Washington ("U-Dub"). The only contact was the association between the head of general medicine in Johannesburg, Professor Tom Bothwell, and the head of hematology at the "U-Dub". Google was years in the future. There was no easy way to get detailed information about the school, its faculty, or facilities, apart from a promotional brochure.

Trusting Tom Bothwell, I took it on faith that there was an acceptable training program in pathology. Unbeknownst to me, this young school, located in a small city on the northwest edge of the continent, had attracted many outstanding faculty. Young turks, progressive and rebellious members of established medical schools, stifled by the academic hierarchy, migrated west for the opportunity to build their careers and their own programs. Build they did. Department after department was lead by world class physician-scientists — from Clement Finch in hematology, to internationally renowned endocrinologist Robert Williams, who was followed by Robert Petersdorf as department chairmen of medicine. Edwin Krebs (biochemistry) and Donnal Thomas (transplantation biology) became Nobel laureates. Henry Harkins built the surgery department. In pathology Karl and Ingegerd Hellstrom were researching the role of the immune system in cancer, fifty years ahead of their time. Within each department, creative faculty were changing the face of medicine. Belding Scribner developed the shunt allowing people to survive renal failure by receiving dialysis. His colleague, Robert Hickman developed an indwelling catheter permitting the easy administration of drugs, as well as being useful for taking samples of blood. The catheter still bears his name.

The energy and intellectual vibrancy of the medical school was palpable. I had moved from an environment of physician-teachers to one of exceptional physician-scientists. It was the epitome of what American medical schools hoped to produce. All organizations go through cycles and I was fortunate to arrive near the zenith of one of these cycles.

The children's hospital, known at the time as Children's Orthopedic hospital, began with seven

176

beds in 1907 to care for children with orthopedic problems. This name endured for years, long after it was managing all childhood diseases. Although a private hospital, its affiliation with medical school grew until it became the pediatric teaching hospital for the university, and all the physicians held academic appointments.

When I joined children's hospital in 1974, the number of full time physicians was so small that we could all gather around a couple of tables at lunchtime. It had the atmosphere of a family. While few in number, many of the medical staff were nationally prominent. Jack Hartman and Ron Chard, both hematologists, joined with colleagues at other major children's hospitals to tackle the tragedy of childhood cancers, especially leukemia. The Children's Cancer Study Group pooled their results and used standard protocols to treat certain tumors. Outcomes for these children improved dramatically. It became a model for pediatric cancer care. The hospital was the epicenter for research on the scourge of the Sudden Infant Death Syndrome. Bruce Beckwith in pathology and George Ray in infectious disease played major roles, enhanced by the inimitable Abe

Bergman, whose political activism led to a number of pieces of life saving legislation for children.

The study and management of birth malformations was another major focus, attracting a group of superstars. Dr. Joseph Warkany, the grandfather of dysmorphology (malformations) spent months in Seattle every year escaping the allergens in the midwest. Together with David Smith, Tom Sheppard, Ron Lemire, David Shurtleff and Bruce Beckwith, the group trained the next generation of dysmorphologists. Once a month we gathered at one of the faculty homes for beer and pizza, to critique the research or presentations of the dysmorphology fellows. This is where we first heard of many of the breakthroughs about some causes of human malformations, such as alcohol. Although the setting was relaxed and informal, the comments and suggestions were insightful. The fellows never gave scientific presentations without the prior sanction of this group.

Sitting at the feet of these intellectual giants, I was at the apogee of pediatric medical science. All of this occurred by happenstance.

Serendipity smiled on me once again — being in the right place at the right time.

Chapter 34. Residency

My first experience in pathology was at University Hospital, on the south side of the University of Washington campus. I soon discovered a couple of soul mates in the residency program. Because of our backgrounds, there was a natural affinity, each of us being outsiders. I was the foreign graduate, generally regarded as a lower form of life, another was black, and the third had come from an osteopathic school, just a notch above an alien. We became good friends.

Over time, we integrated into the mainstream. The chairman of the department took a special interest in me, so I felt supported and comfortable. It also helped that the three of us were pretty good residents. A month into the program I attended a lecture by the pathologist from the children's hospital on "how to perform a pediatric autopsy." It was brilliant. At the end of it I knew exactly the direction my career would take. I scheduled an appointment with him, requesting to work with him at the end of my residency. He looked at me as if I was mildly bonkers and said, "You are just getting started. You have no idea what your interests will be in four years.

We don't even have a training program in pediatric pathology." "No matter," I said, knowing full well that that was my future path.

The strength of the residency at the University of Washington was its variety and diversity of experiences, exposing us to many different practices and teachers. From the private hospital "meat factory", which churned though a huge volume of patients each day; the county hospital with an autopsy room on a upper floor with a 360 degree view of Mt. Rainier, the Olympic mountains, Puget Sound and the Cascades — a novel change from the usual basement location of most morgues; the Public Health hospital — now occupied by Amazon; children's hospital, and the one that I was not permitted to enter, the Veterans Hospital. Being a foreigner they reckoned that I would steal state secrets about government health care. I did not protest, as I saw more than my share of prostate biopsies, lung cancers and cirrhosis at the other institutions.

The best teaching occurred in the private hospital — superb pathologists; an overwhelming volume of material covering the entire spectrum of pathology. The highlight was the director of the laboratory. After the first day on the surgical pathology bench, my draft reports came back to me from his desk covered in red ink. He was the only person who really taught us how to write a succinct and cogent report, and to communicate clearly with the surgeons. These were long, intense and stimulating days.

Following two years of surgical and autopsy pathology, I moved to the Department of Laboratory Medicine, where I found a natural affinity. For one of my rotations, I elected to spend three months in virology, as it was located in Children's Hospital, knowing that I would interact with the staff there. Things went well, as did my research project of developing a simple and rapid test to diagnose herpes infections. I presented the findings at a national microbiology conference in Tucson. As I left the podium I was offered a half dozen jobs in the diagnostic industry. The University of Arizona approached me to head up their virology program. I declined telling them that I wanted to spend more time with the virologist at Children's. So instead of me, they hired him, and I never got the opportunity I was hoping for.

Fortunately the director of pathology at Children's Hospital in Seattle agreed to take me on as a a staff member for the princely salary of $18,000 a year, a small raise from our residency stipend. I was lucky. There were no other pathology positions in Seattle at the time, and all my colleagues had to look elsewhere. Soon after signing a contract, I received a call from a general hospital in Las Vegas. Evidently I had been recommended to them. They were offering a starting salary of $170,000 a year, ten fold higher than I would get in Seattle. I mentioned this to Vivien. "Why don't we go there? You will be able to retire after a couple of years, and then you can do anything you want." "I would not survive that long," I said. "With that amount of money, I would be forced to buy a fast car, drink too much, maybe even gamble, and probably have a mistress or two. Plus I would hate the work. It's not how I envision my life."

The next forty years were spent in children's hospitals, thirty of them in Seattle, and the final ten in Fort Worth, Texas. I have never regretted the decision for a second, although I might have enjoyed driving a Ferrari around the Las Vegas Strip.

Chapter 35. Sudden Infant Death Syndrome (SIDS)

As a freshly minted pathologist, I was thrilled to accept a staff position at the children's hospital in Seattle. Jobs were few and far between at that time and most of my colleagues had to find work in other states. The economy was in a tailspin, and Boeing, one of the largest employers in the region, led the downturn. A sign appeared on the freeway; "Will the last person to leave Seattle please turn out the lights."

When I met with my new boss, he made three announcements; "Firstly," he said, "I take off every Wednesday. That's my steelhead fishing day. You can take off any other day of the week to do as you please. Secondly, we are responsible for performing all the autopsies on babies with suspected sudden infant death. This is an arrangement we have with the county medical examiner, who has deputized us for this purpose. You have to call the family immediately after the autopsy, discuss the findings with them, answer all their questions, and arrange contact with the hospital's SIDS counselors and support group. Finally, I will be out of town for the next three or four months. Now that you are here, I can take the time to attend meetings, testify in medico-legal cases and give presentations to various groups."

This is known as the sink-or-swim approach, also called baptism by fire. I hit the ground running, actually scrambling to stay on two feet without falling. Fortunately, I was able to sit in on some SIDS counseling sessions my boss had with parents before he left town. His skill and empathy were amazing and I soon felt confident enough to fly solo.

One never knew how parents were going to respond when they received the phone call about the autopsy findings. Some were easier than others, but all were emotionally draining. And then there were cases one never forgets.

We received a call from an outlying suburban hospital about a woman who had arrived in their ER with a dead two-month old, suspected to have succumbed to SIDS. The body was transported to us. The next morning I performed the autopsy. Unfortunately, neither the nursing staff nor social workers had bothered to speak to me before I called the mother. I introduced myself and then launched into my standard spiel about SIDS — we don't know the cause; there was nothing you could have done to prevent it; don't blame yourself; there were no other diseases or abnormalities; your baby was obviously well cared for; etc. etc. It was about a fifteen minute talk, after which I invited questions.

The phone was quiet for a moment and then a voice in broken English with a Korean accent said, "What you talking about? You killed baby!! Baby was alive this morning! You killed baby!" I was unprepared for this accusation. It escalated further. "I send friends to shoot you. You kill my baby!" Sobbing and further accusations followed, including being threatened with retribution by one of the Asian gangs from the south side of Seattle.

I called the SIDS social worker to alert her to this problem. "Oh, Dr. Benjamin, weren't you informed that the mother was a little distraught yesterday? In fact she insisted on spending the night in a hospital bed with her dead baby. We had to pry the infant away from her in the morning." "Thanks," I said, "it would have been nice to have had a heads-up."

For the next couple of weeks, I avoided parking my car in the doctors parking lot and was constantly looking over my shoulder. Fortunately, the gang never materialized.

The next threat was more serious. This time I had an excellent conversation with the mother, who appreciated all the information. The father of the baby was in the Navy, onboard a ship in the Pacific, a hundred or so miles offshore. He was to be airlifted to Seattle to attend the funeral. The Navy requested that I speak to him. They patched him through. I proceeded to tell him the same thing I had told the mother. "Dr. Benjamin, I don't believe the diagnosis. I think that you are covering for my girlfriend and that she killed our baby. She smothered the baby because she didn't want to marry me. You are lying to protect her. She killed our baby." "No, sir", I said. "Your baby died of SIDS, I am sorry. Your girlfriend had nothing to do with it." I thought that I was pretty convincing, commiserated with his loss, and left the door open to future questions.

Two days later there was a call from the Military Police. The father had arrived in Seattle and was overheard saying that he was going to kill the doctor who did the autopsy on his child. He was seen leaving the navy base armed with an automatic rifle, heading to Children's Hospital. This set of a conniption. Military Police arrived in force to guard the roads and entrances into the hospital. The security department sent a detail to my office for my personal protection. All quieted down once the father was apprehended upon arrival. I never learned of the final fate of this disturbed young man. I had dodged a potential crime of passion.

One case had a more pleasant outcome. A woman called whose baby had been autopsied more than two decades previously. We talked about SIDS, what had been learned over the past twenty years, some of the latest theories, but I gathered from her tone that something was still bothering her. Finally she said, "All these years I have had nightmares about the autopsy and especially the morgue. I have imagined awful scenes." "Why don't you come to the hospital and I will show you the autopsy suite," I suggested.

She arrived a week later. One could sense her fear, trepidation and apprehension. We chatted for a while, until she was a little more relaxed. Then I led her to the autopsy room in the basement. Upon opening the door a look of relief flooded over her. "It's just like a regular operating room," she said.

For twenty-five years she had lived with an unfounded horror. When she finally garnered the courage to confront the reality, she realized that the ghoulish dread never existed, except in her imagination.

Chapter 36. The Muslim and the Jew

As the quiet Saturday afternoon merged towards dusk, my pager began its raucous beeping. My pulse and blood pressure rose, as pathology emergencies were few and far between. The usual call was to perform a frozen section on a minute fragment of infant gut in order to determine the presence or absence of nerve cells. This disorder, named Hirschsprung's disease, after an obscure Danish physician, produced severe constipation in infants. If not treated promptly, it was potentially fatal. If there was any skill for which we truly earned our pay, this was it — examining a tiny biopsy of a newborn's rectum. This procedure was always a challenge, and a mistake could not just be embarrassing, it could be disastrous. But this call was not to come in to do a frozen section.

The paging operator connected me to the emergency room. A nurse answered. "Dr. Benjamin, we have admitted a family with a dead baby. Looks like a probable case of Sudden Infant Death Syndrome." Feeling relieved that it was not a dire emergency for me, albeit a terrible tragedy for the parents, and knowing that we had dinner plans that evening, I said, "Okay. Have them sign the autopsy permission form, and let them know that I will examine the baby first thing in the morning. I will call them by noon with the results." It was my habit to complete such cases as soon as possible so that the parents would get prompt results, counseling and support.

A half hour later the nurse called me back. "Dr. Benjamin, the parents have refused permission for the autopsy." " Well let them know that by law an autopsy will have to be performed. If we don't do it, then the body will have to be transferred to the medical examiner's office downtown. It may take many days, and they don't have the same resources and counseling service that we have at the children's hospital. Try to convince them that we are the much better option." An hour passed, before the nurse called back to say that the family had finally agreed to allow us to do the examination. I was relieved, but that was short lived.

The nurse was soon back on the phone. "The mother insists on sleeping in the morgue overnight next to the baby." None of us considered this a prime idea. A half dozen phone calls later and the situation was slowly getting resolved. "The mother has agreed to go home, but wants to see the baby again in the morning before the autopsy. And by the way the mother is a Black Muslim, and the father is a Nigerian and a Christian."

"Let's contact the Black Muslim community and try to get a minister to come to the hospital in the morning," I told the nurse. "Also arrange for the hospital chaplain to be there, and we will all meet in the chapel for a viewing." "Oh, one last thing Dr. Benjamin, the mother insists on being present during the autopsy." Never before had I received such a request and I was unprepared to deal with it. " We will discuss it tomorrow", I said, hoping that during the night I would divine some strategy to avoid it. I did not sleep well that night.

At nine o'clock Sunday morning, I met the family in the small, quiet hospital chapel. The early sun shone through the one stained-glass window. The hospital chaplain and a representative of the Black Muslim community were there. The mother was exquisitely statuesque, frighteningly calm and composed. Her husband looked like an professional basketball center. The nursing supervisor entered with the baby, a little girl beautifully swaddled in a fluffy pink blanket, and handed her to the mother. I was still non-plussed with the thought of having her with me during the autopsy. I had not yet developed a plan to avoid it. After some moments of silence with her baby in her arms, she said, "Doctor, during the night I decided that it is fine for you to be alone with my baby, but I do want to prepare the body for the examination and then dress her afterwards." A quiet sigh of relief.

A half hour later, mother and baby were escorted to the autopsy room, while the rest of the entourage departed. The mother gently placed her baby on the polished stainless steel table and undressed her. She then took my hands and began to pray — a Black Muslim woman entrusting her offspring to a white South African Jew. I had goosebumps and choked back tears. Surreal does not do justice to the scene.

The mother left the room, and I began the examination. The findings were typical of Sudden Infant Death - a previously healthy three month old, with scattered hemorrhages on the thymus gland and surface of the lungs, but no other pathology. I worked quickly and sutured the infant with stitches that a plastic surgeon would have been proud of. The mother came back in carrying perfume and oils and a white lace dress. As she was oiling her baby she looked at me and said, "But she is empty." " I thought that you understood that we remove all the organs so that we can examine them under the microscope," I said. "Couldn't you just take small little pieces? I want to be able to bury all of her," she said. "Certainly," I replied. The mother left the room, while I retrieved all the organs, took tiny snippets for microscopic examination, replaced the rest and redid my suturing.

The mother returned, prepared and dressed the body. We left the morgue and together with the father sat in the chapel for an hour, where I told them everything I knew of SIDS, which was pretty much everything that anybody knew at the time. We established contact with the SIDS counsellors and parents-support group and made sure that the couple could contact me in the future with questions. We set a time for a follow-up conference. I left the hospital completely drained, somewhat resembling a damp dishcloth.

During the ensuing months, I received calls from the mother asking if something in her might have been responsible for SIDS. This was an extremely common concern with SIDS parents who perseverate on all the details in their lives and pregnancy prior to the death, seeking a plausible explanation. This mother's questions ran the gamut: could it have been the antibiotics she took for a cold? or the local anesthetic for a dental procedure? Assuaging guilt in mothers is a critical component of SIDS counseling, assuring them that they are not to blame.

About eighteen months later the mother called again, asking if some cryptic or unrecognized disease in the mother might be the cause of the baby's death. I could hear a waver in her voice and asked, "Tell me what you are concerned about." "I have just been diagnosed with acute myeloid leukemia."

A month later she died.

Epilogue - Then and Now

Over fifty years ago, as an eager young medical student, I recall a lecturer telling us that half of what we had just learned would be proven to be wrong. "The problem," he said, "is you don't know which half." He knew what he was talking about. What he failed to mention, was that in fifty years almost everything that one learned in certain areas would be irrelevant.

The fundamentals have remained largely unchanged – anatomy, physiology, pathology and clinical diagnosis. When I recently discarded my medical school notes, I was impressed at how current and pertinent those topics still were. But new diagnostic methods and almost all of therapeutics became unimaginable. New technology has transformed many specialties from which we all benefit.

Even more than these, the entire health care system has changed. The cost of care has far outpaced inflation; the bureaucracy of the insurance industry and the corporatization of medical practice has distanced patients from doctors. Few are satisfied with the current status. Whether the benefits outweigh the downside is for you to decide.

Then: A hernia repair meant a one-week stay in hospital and cost $100.
Today: A hernia repair is an outpatient procedure, you are back at work the next day and it costs $7000.

Then: Only VIPs had private rooms.
Today: There are only private rooms.

Then: To image the brain we filled the head with air, took X-rays and squinted at shadows.
Today: CTs, MRIs and PET scans, now find numerous things, some of which are probably normal.

Then: A kidney transplant was a newsworthy event.
Today: Kidney, liver, heart, pancreas, lung. and assorted body parts are standard. Today only a lopped off penis merits a news flash.

Then: A delivery of a healthy infant was rewarded with 10 days of rest and recreation in hospital.

Today: A delivery is more likely to be an operation, and the modern superwoman requires only 48 hours for full recovery.

Then: Breast cancer meant loss of vast amounts of healthy tissue.
Today: Breast cancer means temporary loss of hair.

Then: Children with leukemia stood a 95% chance of not celebrating their next birthday.
Today: A child with leukemia has an 80% chance of going to college and living long enough to get another cancer.

Then: No one had ever heard of problems with hospital security, apart from the theft of morphine or a few aspirins.
Today: The hospital security staff numbers twice of the number of neonatologists.

Then; Lawyers practiced in fancy offices downtown.
Today; There are as many on-site attorneys as pathologists, and they are more frequently consulted.

Then: Tonsils were removed because they were there.
Today: Tonsils are removed because they are there.

Then: We vaccinated against smallpox and polio.

Today: Small pox is now a terrorist weapon and we no longer require vaccination.Today's vaccines have eliminated most childhood diseases, and *Hemophilus influenzae* meningitis is a distant memory.

Then: Almost every bug responded to penicillin and streptomycin.

Today: Almost no bacterium is sensitive to pen and strep.

Then: Doctors held the hands of terminally ill patients.

Today: Doctors could lose their license if they held the hand of any patient.

Then: Thymuses were irradiated because they were thought to be too big.

Today: Thymuses are removed because they are in the way of the heart surgeon.

Then: A blood transfusion was whole blood, packed red cells or plasma.

Today: A blood transfusion may be one of 42 different products, including, washed, leuco-reduced, irradiated type-specific platelets proven to lack bacterial contamination, every hepatitis virus known to man, HIV, prions, malaria and even syphilis (heaven forbid). Now we know what all those hospital attorneys do for a living.

Then: A doctor made a house call within hours after being summoned.
Today: You have to wait three months to see a physician's assistant half way across town.

Then: No one went bankrupt because of an illness.
Today: Healthcare costs are the major cause of personal bankruptcy.

Then: The doctor was the last person to get paid.
Today: The doctor demands payment before you walk out the door.

Then: Physicians took a complete history and did a thorough physical examination.
Today: Physicians check little boxes on a computer screen and order laboratory tests and X-rays. The stethoscope is a symbol, not a tool.

Then: Blood pressure was measured with a mercury manometer and a stethoscope; the pulse with a watch and temperature with a thermometer.

Today: All these are measured digitally. Nobody knows if they are correct. Mercury is banned (especially in California).

Then: Watches kept track of time.

Today: Watches keep track of your exercise, your sleeping habits, and your heart rhythm.

Then: Physicians had fewer therapeutic options, but really cared about their patients.

Today: Physicians have many therapeutic options, but the health care system inhibits caring.

Then: When in hospital you knew who your doctor was, and saw him/her a couple of times a day.

Today: Your care will be transferred to someone different every eight hours. You will never learn their names.

Acknowledgements

The genesis for recounting these stories was a result of a project begun by a class-mate, Gladwyn Leiman and completed by another, Keith Kaye, to celebrate the 50th anniversary of our medical school class. This project resulted in an avalanche of resumes, recording the careers of an extraordinary group of doctors, all of whom had benefitted from a unique educational and training experience — the University of Witwatersrand Medical School in the 1960's. This narrative is in honor of them and their legendary teachers.

These stories would never have been possible without countless teachers, colleagues, friends and family. It is not feasible to thank each by name.

I chose not to include the names of fellow students in the narrative to protect the innocent. The guilty know who they are. I am however very grateful to Dr. Merlyn Sayers, Dr. Ajit Alles, Hollace Weiner and Mary Kellogg who read portions of the manuscript, providing valuable suggestions. My wife Vivien is a an excellent critic of my writing and although I don't always respond graciously to her suggestions, she is invariably correct. The errors and omissions are my sole responsibility.

www.ingramcontent.com/pod-product-compliance
Lightning Source LLC
Chambersburg PA
CBHW030108300326
41934CB00034B/621